What others say about this book:

"**This book is well overdue.** It addresses a complex subject in a way that will educate the public and health providers. It lays out connections between the jaws and the rest of the body clearly. Chapter headings make it easy to find your way around." —**Dr. Helen Jones, England, U.K.**

"**Both the general public and all health care providers need to read this book** to have a better appreciation and understanding of wellness and total health." —**Dr. Brian Palmer, Kansas City, MO, USA**

"**This publication is an outstanding over view of maxillofacial orthopedics for the patient, the dentist and the physician.**" —**Dr. J. W. "Skip" Truitt, Guadalajara, Mexico**

"**This text concept is long overdue. The public has a right to know about alternatives.** The future lies in medical dentistry concepts. More and more evidence in the scientific literature shows how important jaws are to health and wellbeing. The role of interceptive orthodontic dental treatment in the management of common medical disorders such as bedwetting, snoring, headaches, and middle ear infections cannot be underestimated." —**Dr. Derek Mahony, Sydney, Australia**

"**Very well done! Real-life stories lend drama and interest** to help readers understand the comprehensive health benefits of dental-facial orthopedic care. This is a very positive step in the dissemination of knowledge to the public, about a complex disease syndrome." —**Dr. Jeffrey H. Ahlin, Gloucester, MA, USA**

"**Wow! What a great book!** It provides details ＿＿＿＿ w that are critical for speech-language pathologists and ＿＿＿＿'s to consider. The importance of the jaw in the pr＿＿＿ng, and speaking is frequently underestimat＿＿＿ ＿＿＿ weak jaw can keep the lips and tongue ＿＿＿" —**Diane Chapman Ba＿＿＿, MD, USA**

"**An incredible job.** I will have ＿＿＿ room for patients. I can't begin to imagine the amou＿＿＿ ＿as gone into this book. The FJO chapter is excellent." — ＿＿＿i Yerkes, Woburn MA, USA*

"**An excellent compilation of the current benefits of Functional Jaw Orthopedics.** It should be mandatory reading for all parents, healthcare practitioners and third party providers." —**Richard W. Greenan, Peach Tree City, GA, USA**

"This work is a unique resource for anyone who seeks health and wellness. Dr. Page has masterfully created an interesting, informative and enlightening book. Every sufferer of craniofacial pains, parent or parent-to-be, medical and dental professional should read, understand and share this knowledge."
—Dr. Robert L. Talley, Norman, OK, USA

"Clinical experience and published research cast a light for all to con-template in the area of craniofacial growth, development and diagnosis. I hope that western medicine can expand its focus in order to experience some of the profound benefits functional jaw orthopedics has to offer dental medicine."
—Dr. Warren F. Green, Boston, MA, USA

"This book is as provocative as it is true. The more these ideas spread the better off will be both doctor & patient. Concepts in this book changed my health and my life."
—Dr. Michael S. Bubon, Waukesha, WI, USA

"May this book help speed up a closer relationship between medicine and dentistry. It offers to both patient and health professional alternative care concepts related to jaw imbalance. Symptoms involving the head, ears, heart, airways, face, tonsils and adenoids to mention a few, are found to be part of this total picture." —Dr. Harold Gelb, New York, NY, USA

"This book changes the way we look at jaw to jaw relationships. It clearly demonstrates the correlation between an improper jaw position to such things as headaches, ear problems and even bed-wetting. This book helps unravel the mystery of temporo-mandibular joint dysfunction, one of the most misdiagnosed human disorders. Information presented in this book will enhance the knowledge base of both patients and medical practitioners."
—Tracy Isaacson, B.S, Minneapolis MN, USA

"I hope this book helps others as much as the concepts have helped my daughter and me! I have been providing Functional Jaw Orthopedics to my patients for over 10 years. When it was apparent my daughter would need FJO therapy, I sought to learn more about Dr. Page's early treatment concepts."
—Dr. Steven Fink, Hamburg, NJ, USA

"A great book for patients, parents and medical/dental professionals. This book exposes the cause of many of the most baffling and frustrating childhood health problems, improper jaw development. It is well researched, and it documents the most advanced concepts of "wellness" that the proper jaw relationships—including the TMJ and teeth—provide. Negative effects of airway obstruction, the subsequent abnormal facial growth and development, are presented in a comprehensive and easy to understand manner." —Dr. David B. Miller, Roseville, CA, USA

Your Jaws - Your Life

Alternative Medicine
by David C. Page, D.D.S.

"Truth is stranger than fiction..."

Mark Twain (1835-1910) [1]

"Men occasionally stumble over the truth,
but most of them pick themselves up
and hurry along
as if nothing had happened."

Sir Winston Churchill (1874-1965) [2]

In Appalachia, more than 33% of the elderly
people have lost all their teeth—the highest rate
in a survey of 46 U.S. states.

Centers for Disease Control—1999 [3]

In Appalachia, the burden of coronary heart
disease is greater than in the entire United States.

Morbidity and Mortality Weekly Report—1998 [4]

Your JAWS
Your LIFE

Alternative Medicine

David C. Page, D.D.S.

SmilePage^{SM} Publishing
PO Box 20300
Baltimore, Maryland 21284

Your Jaws - Your Life

Alternative Medicine
by David C. Page, D.D.S.

Published by:
SmilePage^{SM} Publishing
PO Box 20300
Baltimore, Maryland 21284 U.S.A.
Orders@SmilePage.com
http://www.SmilePage.com

Library of Congress Control Number: 2002092657

1st Edition: January 2003

Printed in the United States of America
by Central Plains Book Manufacturing www.centralplainsbook.com

Library of Congress Cataloging-in-Publication Data
Page, David C.
Your jaws your life: alternative medicine/ by David C. Page, D.D.S.

Includes endnote bibliographical references.
ISBN 0-9717368-1-2 Paperback
ISBN 0-9717368-4-7 Hardcover
1. Alternative Medicine—Medical Dentistry
2. Functional Jaw Orthopedics—Jaws
3. Orthodontics & Orthopedics
4. Disease – Airway, Bed-Wetting, Ears, Headaches, Heart

Cover Design by www.TheBookProducer.com
Cover Illustration by Joy Marlowe, M.A., C.M.I.
Cover Quote by Miguel de Cervantes: Don Quixoti, 1605

Unassigned quotations are by David C. Page, D.D.S.

Unless otherwise indicated, all Scripture quotations are taken from the Holy Bible, New Living Translation, Copyright © 1996. Used by permission of Tyndale House Publishers, Inc., Wheaton, Illinois 60189. All rights reserved.

Dedication

This book is dedicated to my dentist predecessors, Dr. Charles L. Page, Sr., and Dr. Charles L. Page, Jr.; to my family—my personal support group; to my staff and my peers—my professional support group who practice Functional Jaw Orthopedics against the odds; to the professionals and patients who have been my consultants and motivators; and to God—my inspiration, who gives all of us The Breath of Life, to pass through Your Jaws ~ Your Life.

Proceeds

A portion of the proceeds from this book will be used by the author to educate health care providers about the wonderful benefits of Functional Jaw Orthopedics (FJO), and to help protect the rights of dental clinicians to practice newer FJO treatment. Patients deserve to have alternative health care choices and alternative care benefits.

"Knowledge is of two kinds.
We know a subject ourselves,
or we know where we can
find information upon it."

Samuel Johnson (1709-1784) [5]

Small Superscript Numbers Denote End Note References

Your Jaws ~ Your Life
Contents

**"Curiosity
is one of the most permanent
and certain characteristics
of a vigorous intellect."**

Samuel Johnson (1709-1784) [6]

**"By fashion we have been taught
that the causes of medical and surgical
diseases are known; yet in reality
very little was understood about
disease until recently, and we still
operate in a scientific twilight."**

**"We have worked with myths
inventing scientific explanation to
cover our lack of knowledge
about the causative factors in illness,
and we have traditionally examined
physiologic organ systems
from a fragmented perspective."**

Clinical Chest Medicine—1980 [7]

Preface: A Note to the Reader

Your Jaws ~ Your Life is designed for easy learning and arranged for use as a health reference. It explains how the teeth and jaws affect overall health.

Modern medicine has made great advances over the past century. But many illnesses are still only managed, as in "managed care." We need real preventive medicine and real "cure-care." Medical dentistry may contribute to better body health for those individuals where treatment is indicated.

The unexplored world of medical dentistry is introduced in this book, which explains the importance of your jaws to your airway and your health. This book teaches how conservative jaw treatments can offer safe, effective and preventive alternative medical care for people of all ages.

You will learn how to carefully explore vast medical databases so you can find out more about your ills. You will also learn how and where to seek providers of unique alternative dental medicine—Functional Jaw Orthopedics—not taught in most dental or medical schools.

Medical dentistry has been missed, dismissed and overlooked, and you should know what it means to you.

Many medical references are listed in the endnotes for you to use when you consult with your healthcare providers.

This book could potentially change and/or extend your life. It can help prepare you to make some wise critical medical care choices for yourself and for those you love.

Your Jaws ~ Your Life may save you time, money and pain. Future medical dentistry may help you live healthier, happier and even longer.

"It is the close observation of little things
which is the secret of success
in business, in art, in science
and in every pursuit in life."

"Human knowledge
is but an accumulation of small facts,
made by successive generations of men,
the little bits of knowledge and experience
carefully treasured up and growing at length
into a mighty pyramid."

Samuel Smiles (1812-1904) [8]

"Seven years of silent inquiry are needful for a
man to learn the truth, but fourteen in order to
learn how to make it known to his fellowmen."

Plato (400 B.C.) [9]

Prologue:
The Author's Short Story

My interest in the jaws (upper and lower) began long before 1980, when I became one of the first third-generation dentists to graduate from the world's first dental school: the Baltimore College of Dental Surgery.

I had a Doctor of Dental Surgery degree at the age of 25. As a new dentist, I had the desire to practice the best general dentistry I knew how–just like my father and grandfather. Fortunately, I was able to treat and observe thousands of patients right away in my father's established practice. I also learned from his vast clinical experience.

My interest in teeth and jaws started early, as I saw how they work together. I learned how to stop my 10 plus years of morning headaches with special orthodontic and orthopedic jaw techniques not taught in dental school.

My interest in smiles and faces grew as I saw how much orthodontic treatment results varied. I learned that after-treatment smiles and faces differed greatly depending upon the treating dentist and their particular approach.

My interest in ears began in 1986, when I saw how my middle son's chronic right ear problems related to his right dental cross-bite. When ear tubes were suggested, I fixed his bite using dental bonding at age 3. His string of 20 consecutive ear problems stopped immediately.

My interest in overall health grew daily as clinical observations brought already published research alive. For two decades, I have searched the medical literature, finding volumes of published research that support my observations. **Your Jaws** can greatly influence the quality of **Your Life**.

**"New opinions
are always suspected,
and usually opposed,
without any reason but because
they are not already common."**

John Locke (1632-1704) [10]

**"There is nothing permanent
except change."**

Heraclitus (500 B.C.) [11]

**"There is danger in reckless change;
but greater danger in blind conservatism."**

Henry George (1839-1897) [12]

Warning-Disclaimer

This book provides a new, simple view of some complicated human health subjects. Many of the topics covered have entire medical texts and specialties devoted to their study. Therefore, only limited amounts of information can be presented.

Many human diseases are multi-factorial, meaning many factors are involved in causing or prolonging disease. So remember, there is no single way to prevent, diagnose or treat every human disease. However, you should find priceless useful treasures for you and your loved ones in **Your Jaws ~ Your Life.**

This text provides information in regard to the subject matter covered. It is sold with the understanding that the publisher and author are not engaged in rendering medical or other professional services. If medical or other expert assistance is required, the advice and services of a competent professional should be sought.

Alternative medical treatment discussed in this book is based on clinical or research findings current at the time the book was written. Individual treatment results presented are specific to a patient and do not guarantee the same for others.

You are urged to learn as much as possible about any alternative medical treatment of interest to you, utilizing the many references and resources available.

You should consult with your own personal health care providers before starting any therapy described in this book. The publisher and author do not represent or warrant that treatments recommended in this book are medically effective and are not responsible for any adverse effects or consequences resulting from the use of any suggestion or procedure contained in this book.

The publisher and author shall have neither liability nor responsibility to any person or entity with respect to any loss or damage caused, or alleged to be caused, directly or indirectly by the information contained in this book: **Your Jaws ~ Your Life.**

**"Bodies cannot live without abundance of air;
that is, without its being furnished
for inspiration and respiration
in considerable quantity."**

Vitruvius (1ˢᵗ Century B.C.) [13]

**ABCs of CPR:
Opening the airway (A) is one of the first steps in
cardiopulmonary resuscitation (CPR).**

**CPR uses a "head tilt-chin lift" or
"jaw thrust" maneuver to move a jaw forward, in
order to open a closed airway.**

American Heart Association—2000 [14]

**"We must learn to pay closer attention
to the human airway."**

Singapore Medical Journal—2001 [15]

Introduction

For thousands of years we have been searching for the true causes of many common human disorders like bed-wetting, ear disease, headache, hypertension and heart disease. Curiously, the primary causes of some major human disorders may be right under our noses.

Your jaws are as important to your health as your heart and brain. The jaws help determine how long you will live and how healthy you will be. Jaw balance or imbalance affects humans of all ages. Why then are the human jaws ignored throughout most of life until you are sick or dying?

Your airway is ignored one-third of your lifetime, when you sleep. This could be the most important time of all! Snoring is one warning sign your jaws may be affecting you.

Your teeth support your jaws and jaw balance. Teeth preserve tongue space and vital airway breathing space.

A big void in health education may be responsible for a number of chronic human illnesses remaining uncured. Medical and dental schools do not generally teach beyond fetal growth how the jaws, airway and teeth all form, function, and deform together throughout life. Consequently, medical doctors and dental doctors get little training in how the complicated jaws, airway and teeth all work together.

A major void in healthcare treatment exists today. Medical doctors pay little attention to the jaws, airway and teeth until a patient needs sedation or cardiopulmonary resuscitation (CPR). Dental doctors generally treat teeth and gums, not the jaws, ears or airway.

Accordingly, chronically sick patients feel forced to seek effective alternative therapies more than ever before.[16]

**The United States is
#1 in spending per person for healthcare but
#24 in longevity (length of life).**

World Health Organization (WHO)—2000 [17]

**"Insanity:
doing the same thing over and over again
and expecting different results."**

Albert Einstein (1879-1955) [18]

**Functional Jaw Orthopedics can be
medically effective,
exceptionally unique and unequaled in speed of a
cure for a number of very common medical
conditions currently only "managed"
by modern medicine.**

The Functional Orthodontist —1999 [19]

Patients are seeking alternative care because of the limitations and high cost of conventional medicine. Most patients want cost-effective treatments that work. Studies show over 50% of the public have already used or plan to use alternative medical therapies. Patients want effective choices.

Some researchers who recognize the limitations of modern medicine are searching the globe for alternatives. As a result some simple ancient remedies are now being used again, even after medicine overlooked and detested them as unthinkable. For example, maggots heal chronic wounds; honey cleans wounds; leeches thin blood; and deep nasal breathing may be a simple way to reverse artery hardening.[20]

An unexplored world of health exists right under the nose. The upper and lower jaws form the gateway to the human airway. It has been reported that small jaw growth puts both newborn infants at risk of dying from Sudden Infant Death Syndrome (SIDS) and adults at risk of dying from heart disease. It was known for decades that packing the nose before surgery would cause mysterious blood gas changes, including drops in oxygen. Not until the late 1990s did researchers discover why this happened. They found that nasal breathing differs greatly from mouth breathing. Inhaling air through the nose is natural chemotherapy.

Good dental care and saving teeth can potentially lead to a healthier, happier and longer life. Once you understand the value of good mouth care, going to your dental doctor (dentist) can be something you actually want to do.

Functional Jaw Orthopedics (FJO) can be effective dental medicine. Dentists who provide FJO treatments need unique knowledge and expert clinical skills. Some of these dentists have dealt with the airway, breathing, bed-wetting, breast-feeding, ear disease, early orthodontics, headaches, heart disease, sleep apnea, snoring, teeth and tonsils and have noted a relationship with jaw problems.

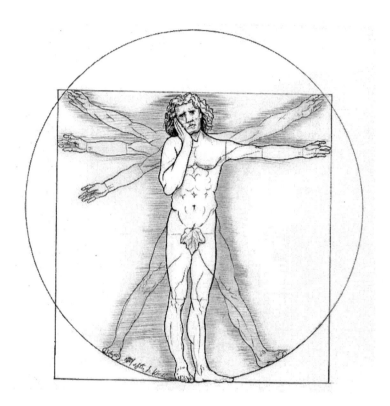

The Jaws Image
Shows The Slow Curse of Modernization

Leonardo da Vinci's "Vitruvian Man"(c.1492)—Revised

The Jaws Image

Leonardo da Vinci was a genius. He was likely the most remarkable artist, scientist and intellectual of the Great Renaissance. You may have seen his famous smiling "Mona Lisa" or "The Last Supper" paintings. Born in 1452 A.D. he was very curious about physical things. His love of knowledge and research led him to keep precise records of his countless ideas, observations and inventions.

Leonardo da Vinci was a great scientific detective. He found overlooked treasures in the writings of 1st century B.C. Roman architect Marcus Vitruvius Pollio. The 1500- year-old writings helped him design hydraulics, machinery and flying machines. Pollio's measurements of the body led da Vinci to illustrate mathematic algorithms and geometric genius in his "Vitruvian Man" drawing. It was only recently discovered how da Vinci brilliantly solved the mathematical problem known as "squaring the circle" in that image.[21]

The Jaws Image, a revised "Vitruvian Man," is designed to show how today, slow degenerative disease continues to occur, in spite of our best efforts. Known as the curse of modernization, this plague on humanity brings diabetes, hypertension, heart disease, and early death to our door, too often and too soon. Degenerative disease happens so slowly, that medical and dental eyes often do not see the relationships between jaws, airways, and related diseases.

The Jaws Image reminds us of how important the overlooked jaws are to general health. The jaws form the gateway to the human airway. Poorly developed or crooked jaws slowly can turn healthy humans into chronically sick ones. Small jaws make small airways. Lack of oxygen can kill fast, or more often slowly and somewhat silently. **Complex modern medicine needs to take a simple look and a new view of the human jaws, airway and body.**

**If he grinds his teeth
the disease will last a long time.**

Sumerian Clay Tablets—3500 to 3000 B.C. [22]

**In that place there will be
weeping and gnashing of teeth.**

Holy Bible [23]

**History records
that physical health and illness
are functions of biological processes and
medical care, along with social, psychological
and behavioral factors.**

Journal of Health and Social Behavior—2002 [24]

**The jaw is a critical
and often ignored structure
in the functions of
eating, drinking, and speaking.**

Oral Motor Assessment and Treatment—2001 [25]

The Jaws & History

As early as 3500 B.C. the Sumerians recorded how the status of teeth related to illness. They used clay tablets to record the diagnostic and treatment protocols of their advanced civilization. Many of the clay tablets later became references as part of the Royal library of Assyrian King Ashurbanipal after 1700 B.C.

Grinding of teeth was seen as a sign of poor health and even impending death. Tooth grinding was considered so serious that the cultural goddess of Ishtar—the mother of life and death—was believed to be involved.

One remedy proposed for grinding of the teeth included putting a human skull on a chair for three days and adding sacrifices to it each morning and night.[26]

Around 1000 B.C. the Hebrews recorded in the Old Testament the high value of healthy teeth. Teeth were regarded as symbols of strength. Tooth loss stood for weakness and sickness. Physical requirements for the high priest included having a whole body and no missing teeth.

The Bible, a worldwide best seller year after year, records the relationship between stress and the grinding of teeth numerous times. Several references are made to stress resulting in **"the weeping and gnashing of teeth."**[27]

History teaches us that what is old is not always bad, or useless, and what is new is not always good, or useful.

In 1951, at the charter meeting of the American Academy of the History of Dentistry, a statement was made that directly applies to and predicts future medical dentistry: **"The only guide to the future is the study of the past."**

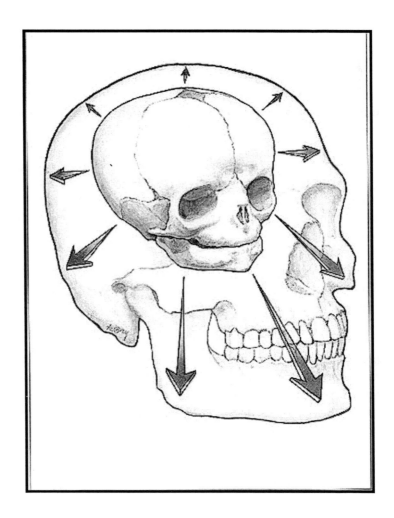

Shaping the Face & Jaws

The challenge of jaw orthopedics is to guide growth of baby
jaws into normal adult jaws, with minimum interference.

Figure and Paraphrased Text Courtesy of Dr. Jeffrey Ahlin
Maxillofacial Orthopedics: A Clinical Approach for the Growing Child

The Jaws & Teeth

The jaws and teeth are essential to human survival. They each have multiple primary roles in sustaining life. Teeth are often overlooked, but they do provide critical jaw and airway support. Jaw support is necessary to maintain tongue space, airway space and basic life support.

Jaws form the gateway to the human airway. The jaws and surrounding structures can affect the airway.

The jaws are taken for granted most of the time. You breathe life-giving air through your jaws. You eat food and drink fluids with your jaws. Jaws can be used as tools. Even kissing involves the jaws. The jaws essentially help you obtain many basic needs and wants in your life. Jaw anatomy is very complex, and so is jaw function.

Human jaws consist primarily of two connected upper jawbones known as the maxilla or palate, and the much larger lower jawbone known as the mandible. Secondarily, the jaws interconnect with all other bones of the skull and neck directly or by way of the many attached muscles, tendons, blood and lymph vessels, and nerves.

Jaws must grow down and forward to form the lower half of a mature human face. Various backward forces on the jaws or teeth prevent proper jaw growth, and can decrease the size of the jaws and then the airway.

Jaw and tooth development continue to about age 30. Breastfeeding, bottle-feeding, swollen tonsils and adenoids, and nasal obstruction influence proper jaw growth and tooth alignment. **Few people have a broad understanding of how these complex processes relate because the many relationships are not generally taught.**

The first year of life,
is the strongest period of jaw growth.

By age 6, about 90% of head growth, and about
80% of jaw growth has already occurred.

Facial Growth and Facial Orthopedics—1986 [28]

Breast suckling can promote proper jaw growth.
Bottle and pacifier sucking can work against it.

The Functional Orthodontist—2001 [29]

The greatest increase in lower jaw
length and width occurs before 9 months of age.

The lower jaw grows twice as fast
as the upper jaw between 1 and 6 years of age.

A small upper jaw
can hold back proper lower jaw growth.

Proper jaw development is
the most critical factor influencing
whether a malocclusion (a bad bite) develops.

Maxillofacial Orthopedics:
A Clinical Approach for the Growing Child—1984 [30]

At birth the upper and lower jaws are flat and only about 30% of their full adult size. The small upper and lower jaws grow to form the lower half of the adult face. The skull forms the upper half of the adult face and is already about 65% of its full size at birth. Skull and brain growth slow after age 4. The jaws continue to grow rapidly allowing the jaws to catch up to the skull by about age 6.

Breast-feeding (suckling) promotes good down and forward jaw growth during a critical period of rapid jaw growth. So exclusive breastfeeding for 3-6 months is crucial and usually best for infant jaws. Breastfeeding has many lifelong health benefits. Better jaws and airways are responsible for some of those benefits.

Bottle-feeding and pacifier use (sucking) prevent proper jaw growth. Early backward forces of sucking deform jawbones, prevent proper growth, cause smaller jaws, and increase dental crowding and malocclusion in modernized cultures. Babies that do not suckle may suffer for life.

By age 6 the jawbones and skull bones normally grow 80-90% of their adult size. So orthodontics at age 8 can be too late to influence proper balanced jaw growth.

Jaws and airways are getting smaller. Diet, infant feeding practices and some orthodontic extraction techniques are key reasons. Comparisons of ancient and modern skulls confirm this change. Most people today have jaws about ¼ inch too small to fit all the wisdom teeth into place. Sadly, small jaws and airways can bring about premature death.

Teeth act like pillars to keep upper and lower jaws apart. Premature tooth loss can cause jaws to collapse.[31] If jaws collapse, tongue and airway space is lost. A tongue can become a deadly choker. The jaws and tongue can drop into the throat and block the airway when sleeping on the back. **Snoring may signal a dangerously blocked airway.**

**"It is the little things—
infected teeth and tonsils, for instance—
that cause most of our serious ailments."**

Dr. Charles H. Mayo—1934 [32]

**Save your teeth and save or extend your life!
Good dental function
is significantly associated with
better brain function,
better vision,
better hearing,
better lung volume,
better heart volume,
better muscle strength,
better bone mineral content,
less heart attacks
and longer life.**

British Medical Journal—1989 [33]
Community Dental Oral Epidemiology—1990 [34]

**"Every tooth in a man's head
is more valuable to him than a diamond."**

Cervantes: Don Quixote—1605 [35]

What did Dr. Charles H. Mayo observe about teeth and tonsils that deserved his direct blame for causing most of our serious ailments? Dr. Mayo was a well-known and well-respected medical authority in the 1900s. He was also one of the founders of the distinguished Mayo clinic. Interestingly, he saw back then what medicine has overlooked for so long. He observed the clinical association between bad teeth and bad health, and the importance of good teeth to good health.

Some say Dr. Mayo went too far to blame "most of our serious ailments" on "teeth and tonsils." Did he? Could it just be that people who have their teeth take better care of themselves in other areas? Or, could it be they just eat better? Dr. Mayo saw what researchers around the world have missed. When teeth are lost and not replaced, general health often declines. Additionally, lifespan can be shortened.

Tooth loss worldwide has been associated with higher rates of human disease and premature death. In the U.S., a map showing regions of highest total tooth loss also shows the regions of greatest health disparities, illness, heart disease and premature death.[36] It is often assumed that those with more teeth are healthier because they take better care of themselves. It may be just as true that those with more teeth have better airways, which keep them healthier.

The first ever U.S. Surgeon General's report on Oral Health was delivered in May of 2000. The report addresses the need to promote better oral health and to research the relationships between oral and general health. The oral health report serves as evidence that we have much to learn about how teeth support the jaws, preserve tongue and airway space, and affect life.

Cervantes penned Don Quixote as a foolish heroic madman. Equating the value of a tooth to a diamond may excuse Quixote's character and at last win him some respect.

**"The first breath
is the beginning of death."**

Thomas Fuller (1732) [37]

**"God formed a man's body
from the dust of the ground
and breathed into it the breath of life."**

Holy Bible (B.C.) [38]

**Proper airway development depends upon
good jaw and facial growth.
Equally, proper jaw and facial development
depends upon good airway growth.**

Essentials of Facial Growth—1996 [39]

**Nasal airway breathing obstruction may result in
craniofacial (skull and jaw) deformities,
if present before or during puberty.**

*American Journal of Orthodontics and
Dento-facial Orthopedics—1997* [40]

The Jaws & Airway (Breathing)

Your jaws form the gateway to your human airway and influence your life, for life. Your jaws are fundamentally as important to your health and survival as your heart and your brain. The airway through which you breathe includes two nose nostrils and the mouth.

Jaws, surrounding structures, and airways differ greatly from person to person. Most people can breathe through the mouth. Some people can breathe well through the nose; others cannot. Some breathe well through one or both nostrils, and others cannot. Breathing pathways influence the ability to get oxygen into the lungs and body.

Humans with larger airways tend to breathe better and they often perform better athletically. You can see this daily if you take a close look at the strong jaws and masculine faces of most professional athletes. They are often big jaw, big airway, and big performance people.

Humans with smaller airways tend to have more breathing problems and thus performance problems. Studies show there is a direct relationship between small upper airway size and asthma, respiratory disorders,[41] obstructive sleep disorders, hypertension, and heart disease. The association is not well known, but it is well documented.

Airways tend to shrink with age. The uvula, tongue, and throat tissues tend to lose tone and become more flaccid over time. **Obesity and age related weight gain** can make things much worse.[42] Obesity causes swelling of the tongue, uvula and throat tissues directly proportional to weight gain.[43]

During sleep, gravity can pull the lower jaw, tongue, uvula and other tissues into the throat. A blocked airway makes a unique choking sound you can hear—snoring.

Nasal airway obstruction has profound effects on the whole body, and can even determine a patient's symptoms and complaints.

Otolaryngologic Clinics of North America—1989 [44]

Nitric oxide (NO) is a gas produced in the paranasal sinuses, excreted continuously into the nasal airways, and inhaled through the nose. It is well known to prevent bacterial growth.

Nature Medicine—1995 [45]

Inhaled NO is a potent lung vasodilator. It increases the lung's ability to absorb oxygen, and therefore it raises blood oxygen levels.

Pediatric Research—1999 [46]

Nasal NO gas is present in healthy newborn infants within the first hour after birth.

Pediatric Research—1996 [47]

Not all snoring is deadly. But frequent loud snoring is a major recognizable sign of a blocked airway. Snoring can be an emergency siren. It usually sends out a signal when someone is in trouble. Yet it may produce a false alarm.

Nasal breathing, breathing through the nose, is now known to be vital to good health. Researchers in the late 1990s, found that mouth-inhaled air does not benefit the lungs and body the same way as air inhaled through the nose.

Inhaling deeply through the nose then exhaling slowly through the mouth has been used for thousands of years to improve health. Although the actual biochemical process of deep nasal breathing was not known until recently, nitric oxide gas inhalation explains a good bit of it.

Nitric oxide (NO) gas was discovered in the nasal passages in the 1990s. Nobel prizes were awarded to researchers who discovered that the body produced NO.

Nitric oxide is a potent gas and a key component of human health. NO is produced in the nasal sinuses, secreted into the nasal passages and inhaled through the nose. In the lungs it improves the ability to absorb oxygen. NO is also produced in blood vessel walls. It is a strong vasodilator and brain transmitter. It increases oxygen transport throughout the body and is vital to all body organs.

Breathing nitric oxide produced by the nose is natural chemotherapy. Nasally inhaled NO can affect the whole body. NO produced in the walls of blood vessels relaxes blood vessels, so it was given the name endothelial relaxation factor-ERF. NO is everywhere in the body and may well control the function of every major body organ system. Researchers discovered that diet affects NO levels. Researchers also know **nitric oxide like oxygen must be in balance, because too much of either gas can be toxic.**

Nitric Oxide (NO) is everywhere in the body.
It plays a role in the function of most organs.
It can kill some bacteria and viruses.
It has anti-inflammatory effects.
It may play a key role in heart disease.
It may play a key role in aging.

Experimental Gerontology—1998 [48]

Nasally inhaled NO has been shown
to increase oxygen exchange by 10%
and to increase blood oxygen by 18%.

Acta Physiologica Scandinavica—1996 [49]

Studies have shown that blocking NO production
in healthy humans results in
moderate hypertension,
reduced heart output,
and shortened bleeding times
by activation of platelet blood-clotting factors.

Acta Anaesthesiologica Scandinavica—1997 [50]

The potent effects of nitric oxide may be evident in millions of homes on a regular basis. Cooking bacon in a closed house increases the levels of nitric oxide in the air. Because nitric oxide is a strong brain transmitter, only tiny amounts are needed to stimulate the brain. That may explain why cooking bacon tends to awaken those who are asleep.

If you cannot breathe through your nose well, you are not getting the enormous benefits of nitric oxide. You should be concerned because you may suffer long-term health consequences. Consider some groups of mouth breathers who cannot regularly breathe well through the nose: those with Marfan's syndrome; Down syndrome; Dwarfism; and the mentally retarded. As a group, these mouth breathers often die prematurely of heart disease.

Research shows mouth breathers get less oxygen, because they do not benefit from inhaled nasal nitric oxide. At the same time they retain more carbon dioxide. This may explain why mouth breathing is harmful to health and IQ.

The short-term effects of mouth breathing were recognized decades ago. Patients who had the nose packed in preparation for surgery would undergo a drop in blood oxygen for unknown reasons. Upon removal of the nasal packing the blood oxygen levels would rise again.

The long-term effects of mouth breathing have only recently been recognized and documented. Mouth breathers tend to have lower levels of blood oxygen and higher levels of carbon dioxide, especially at night. Mouth breathers tend to be sicker and have more heart trouble. They rarely catch up in health or IQ to breastfed infants who are frequently nasal-breathers. Mouth breathing commonly causes crooked teeth (malocclusion). Mouth breathing tends to cause open-bite jaw deformation, which then can negatively affect the airway and overall face.

Mouth breathers
can become nose breathers.

A 1975 study selected 310 patients
between the ages of 4 and 31 to undergo
dental treatment for medical reasons.

Palatal expansion produced phenomenal results.
Palatal expansion (a form of FJO treatment)
widens a narrow palate without drugs or surgery.
It is a comparatively simple and conservative way
of treating impaired nasal respiration.

Study results suggest palatal expansion is medically
indicated for those with a poor nasal airway,
deformed septum, recurrent ear or nasal infection,
allergic rhinitis (runny nose), asthma and those
where septum surgery failed previously.

**Colds, respiratory infections, nasal allergies and
many cases of asthma** also improved considerably
after palatal expansion.

**80% of those who were mouth breathers before
treatment became nasal breathers after only
1 to 3 months of dental treatment.**

The Journal of Laryngology and Otology —1975 [51]

Mouth breathing is fairly preventable and usually treatable if appropriate therapy begins very early.

Exclusive breastfeeding for about 6 months, when possible, helps prevent mouth breathing.

Bottle-feeding and pacifiers promote mouth breathing. Finger sucking, thumb sucking and tongue thrust habits also increase rates of mouth breathing.

Large tonsils and adenoids also force some people to become mouth breathers. Routine tonsil and adenoid removal would help considerably with this health villain.

Early Functional Jaw Orthopedics can widen the mouth to make more room for the tongue and increase the overall airway. **Oral motor and myofunctional therapists** can play key roles in the early correction of mouth breathing.

Mouth breathing that goes unchecked deforms jaws and airways. Improper jaw and airway growth causes jaw and airway deformation and dysfunction. Mouth breathing can affect the face and whole body, and affect them for life.

Nasal airway obstruction that goes unchecked can be a slow killer. It may also cause some sudden deaths.

Simple overnight pulse-oxygen measurement is a way to screen for low blood oxygen levels, known as hypoxia. Unfortunately, overnight pulse-oxygen testing equipment is not yet readily available for general public use. Only an overnight medical sleep study can confirm whether low blood oxygen and a sleep disorder exists.

If you are the parent of a young mouth breather, Functional Jaw Orthopedics provides non-surgical hope for enlarging a small airway and it should be considered. **For those over age 30,** the options are more complicated.

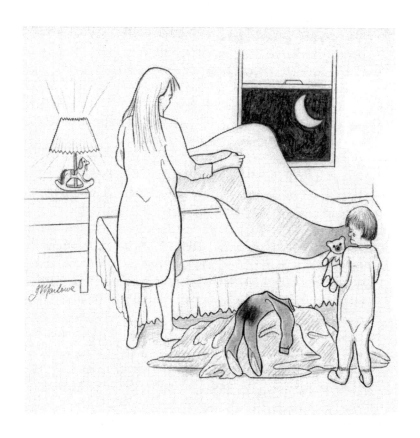

**Despair
exaggerates not only our misery
but also our weakness.**

Luc De Vauvenargues (1746) [52]

**The primary or exact cause
of most bed-wetting remains unknown.**

Pediatric Nephrology—1995 [53]

The Jaws & Bed-wetting
(Nocturnal Enuresis)

Bed-wetting remains a puzzle for modern medicine. It continues to be the most common urologic problem for 5 to 7 million school age children in the U. S. The exact cause of chronic bed-wetting is frequently unknown, so bed-wetting is often "managed" and not cured.[54] **Dental jaw treatment may help some children with this problem.**

Nocturnal enuresis is the medical term for nighttime bed-wetting, or involuntary loss of urine during sleep. The term comes from the Greek word enourein, meaning "in urine" or "inability to control urination."

Normal bladder control should occur by age 3-4. It is considered medically abnormal when a child over age 5 chronically wets the bed. From 15 to 20% of all 5 year-olds and 10% of all 6-10 year-olds chronically wet the bed. For unknown reasons boys do so more than girls.[55]

Bed-wetting causes great psychosocial suffering. It is humiliating, exhausting, embarrassing, and upsetting for the child and other family members. It limits social involvement. It produces major strain and tends to frustrate entire families.[56] In spite of this, some health care providers consider bed-wetting to be a low-severity disorder.

The financial cost of managing bed-wetting is often underestimated.[57] A monthly supply of drugs alone can cost over twice the $100 price of a bed-wetting alarm.[58] Total costs of not treating enuresis (travel, diapers, washing, drying, etc.) can be higher than alternative treatment costs.[59]

Historically the Egyptians recognized bed-wetting as a medical problem in 1550 B.C. Bed-wetting was recorded in the first English-language book for pediatricians.[60]

**Doctors often dismiss nocturnal enuresis—
bed-wetting—as a minor problem and suggest
that the child will 'grow out of it.'**

Nursing Standard—1998 [61]

**All medical approaches to date reflect a lack of
sufficient knowledge of the underlying
true causes of nocturnal enuresis,
commonly known as bed-wetting.**

Clinical Pediatrics—1993 [62]

**Drugs make up a good portion of
bed-wetting treatment although results are less
than desired, and real risks exist.
Bed-wetting relapse occurs at very high rates
once drug therapy ends.**

Clinical Pediatrics—1998 [63]

**Children with ADHD—
Attention Deficit Hyperactivity Disorder—
are 2 1/2 times more likely
to be bed-wetters.**

Southern Medical Journal—1997 [64]

Some very cruel remedies were used to treat chronic bed-wetting. They proved ineffective, acting more like forms of punishment or torture. Old remedies included: tying a string around the child's penis; pouring cold streams of water over the spine; making the child sit on a hot stove; forcing the child to drink a pint of his or her own urine; physician prescribed ingestion of ground-up hedge-hog testicles; and painful cauterization of the urethra with silver nitrate.[65]

Modern medicine has a long list of possible causes of nocturnal enuresis. The list includes genetic inheritance, reduced bladder capacity, sleep disorders, abnormal secretion of an anti-diuretic hormone, psychological abnormalities, neurological dysfunction, bacteria in the urine, and diet.[66]

Current medical treatment approaches may reflect a lack of sufficient knowledge of the underlying true causes of nocturnal enuresis.[67] Some current management options include drugs, bed-is-wet alarms, psychotherapy, electrophysiology, and surgery.[68] The enuresis alarm with behavior reinforcement, the most effective treatment to date, is the least often prescribed.[69] Drugs, the treatment with the strongest scientific research, interestingly may be the least effective. Although often-prescribed demopressin medication appears to have few side effects, there are increasing reports it may be causing hyponatremic (low serum sodium) seizures.[70] [71]

Bed-wetting research has not provided conclusive evidence of the cause of bed-wetting.[72] Research tends to be centered on using prescription drugs, so drugs make up a good portion of bed-wetting therapy. Current medical protocols cannot recommend a successful cure for bed-wetting, because the true cause of most bed-wetting is not known. However, there is new hope and good reason for it.

Dental treatment, although not currently recommended by modern medicine, can be effective in reducing or stopping chronic bed-wetting.

**Adolescents aged 12-16 years,
referred for psychological pathology study,
(depression, ADHD, etc.) were 7 times more
likely to wet the bed than controls.**

Journal of Paediatrics and Child Health—1995 [73]

**Functional Jaw Orthopedics
can turn mouth breathers into nasal breathers,
and is about 80% effective in reducing or
stopping chronic bed-wetting in children in about
one to three months.**

**Published in 1990...10 of 10 chronic bed-wetters
stopped after just a few months of starting
rapid palatal expansion.**

Angle Orthodontist—1990 [74]

**Published in 1998....7 of 10 non-responder
chronic bed-wetters, aged eight to thirteen,
who failed to respond to conventional treatments
improved within one month of rapid
palatal expansion.**

Angle Orthodontist—1998 [75]

A retrospective study published in 1990 looked at the records of 100 children after dental treatment. Ten children were found to be bed-wetters before dental rapid palatal expansion—a form of Functional Jaw Orthopedics that widens the roof of the mouth. All 10 of those chronic bed-wetters stopped after only a few months of treatment.[76]

A prospective study published in 1998 analyzed the effects of rapid maxillary expansion in 10 children between the ages of 8 and 13 called non-responders. Of the 10 bed-wetters who did not respond to conventional medical treatment, 7 improved after maxillary expansion. Of these 7, 4 were dry, and 3 showed improvement in about one month.[77]

Research shows a lack of oxygen due to upper airway obstruction can cause bed-wetting. Reversing the airway obstruction or increasing blood oxygen levels may stop it. Tonsillectomy in children opens airways and reduces bed-wetting.[78][79] Oral devices and forced air oxygen given to adults can help stop bed-wetting. Some children "grow-out-of" bed-wetting as their jaws and airways grow. Early Functional Jaw Orthopedic treatment, which turns about 80% of mouth breathers into nose breathers, can reduce or stop bed-wetting in about 80% of those from ages 4 to 31.

The 1990 and 1998 combined study results show dental treatment to be about 80% effective in reducing or stopping bed-wetting in just a few months.

Dental treatment may be 5 to 7 times more effective than doing nothing to stop bed-wetting, considering only about 15% of bed-wetters spontaneously stop each year.

If you know a bed-wetter, consider getting an FJO checkup. If FJO treatment is needed, a decrease in bed-wetting might be an additional benefit. Research suggests the earlier FJO treatment starts, the more likely it will help.

**During breast suckling,
the undulating rhythmic elevation and lowering
of the jaw stimulates lower jaw growth,
during the most rapid period of jaw growth.**

Handbook of Facial Orthopedics—1982 [80]

**A strong association has been found between
exclusive bottle-feeding and malocclusion.**

Journal of the Canadian Dental Association—1991 [81]

**Research shows children breastfed about 1 year
rarely develop dummy or finger sucking habits.**

Swedish Dental Journal—1998 [82]

**Non-breast sucking habits
such as fingers and dummies (pacifiers)
are strongly associated with
crooked teeth and/or jaws (malocclusion).**

Acta Odontologica Scandinavica—1993 [83]

The Jaws & Breastfeeding

Breastfeeding helps jaws and airways to develop properly. Bottle and pacifier use can deform jaws and airways. Breast **suckling** promotes good forward jaw growth and development. Bottle, pacifier and finger **sucking** put backward forces on the jaws during one of the most important periods of rapid forward growth. **Dentists should advocate breastfeeding for about 6 to 12 months.**

Research shows breastfed infants have considerably less illness and fewer lifelong health problems. Breast-fed babies are less likely to develop allergies, ear infections, insulin-dependent diabetes, respiratory infections, gastrointestinal infections, diarrhea, and lymphomas (a form of cancer). Breast-fed babies are less likely to be hospitalized for serious illness, less likely to die of SIDS, and generally have higher IQs. Recent research found increased intelligence in adults who were breastfed as infants.[84]

Some of the health benefits of breastfeeding are due to better jaw and airway formation, although most credit has been given to the content of a nursing mother's milk. The forward forces of breast suckling cause down and forward growth of the jaws, enlarging the room for the tongue and airway. Backward constricting forces of bottle and pacifier sucking can cause dental malocclusion and jaw deformation, which also can reduce tongue and airway space.

In 1973, only about 26% of new mothers in the U.S. chose to breastfeed. In the 1980s, New Guinea took steps to restrict the use of baby bottles because they saw how diseases such as diabetes, hypertension and heart disease increased as breastfeeding decreased in modernized cultures. Many modern societies are starting to encourage breastfeeding again. **Dentists can help reduce disease and promote better health by advocating infant breastfeeding.**

**Preventive fluoridation of drinking water
reduced tooth decay and tooth loss so effectively
that it was rated 1 of the top 10 major health
accomplishments of the 20th Century.**

Center for Disease Control—1999 [85]

**Dental amalgam
is remarkably durable and long lasting.
Although its appearance is un-esthetic, its clinical
performance and effectiveness are unsurpassed
by those of resin composite.**

Quintessence International—2001 [86]

**This epidemiological study of women found
"no connection between the number of
amalgam fillings and health."**

Lakartidningen (Article in Swedish)—2001 [87]

**A lifespan study of 2,035 fillings found
dental amalgams lasted on average 15 years,
while plastic composites lasted about 8 years.**

The Journal of the American College of Dentists—1998 [88]

**"1,000,000 patients are injured each year
due to medication related problems."**

Prescription Caused Medical Problems—1999 [89]

The Jaws & Dental Care

Until about 150 years ago, dental infection from decayed and abscessed teeth, was a main cause of death. This changed when dentists and dental care became more available and affordable. Treating tooth decay significantly reduced dangerous and deadly dental infections.

For 150 years, dental amalgam fillings have played a key role in treating decayed teeth. Dental amalgam has extended millions of lives worldwide by saving billions of teeth that support the jaws and keep airways open. The safety record of dental amalgam is impressive.[90] In 150 years, no patient death or illness has been recorded as being due to either dental amalgam or dental amalgam mercury except for rare cases of allergy.[91][92] Amalgam is safe, strong, long lasting, effective, and economical.[93][94] Promoting dental amalgam removal for health reasons is deemed unethical.[95][96]

Plastic tooth colored composite filling materials are used frequently now. Some people blame dental amalgam for illnesses with no known cause, and stir fear.[97] Psychological fear drives some patients to replace their amalgam fillings with plastic fillings.[98][99] While plastic composites appear rather safe, some long-term concerns do exist about their shorter lifespan and effects on tissues. [100][101]

Compare the safety of all dental care to prescription drug care. In 1994, an estimated 2,216,000 people in the U.S. had serious legal-drug reactions resulting in hospitalization or permanent disability. Also, 106,000 died of mostly preventable deaths.[102] Legal drugs burden our health care system with 5-15% of hospitalization costs: up to $130 billion annually.[103]

When choosing dental care, patients and doctors should keep in mind the main goal, which is to save teeth, keep jaws supported, and keep the airways open.

Removing complete dentures
during sleep
promotes breathing disorders
and increases both the risk of hypertension
and cardiovascular disease.

Minerva Stomatologica—2000 [104]

* Removing dentures to sleep removes
support for tongue space.
As support for tongue space is lost, the tongue
goes into the throat during sleep.
The tongue blocks the airway, which blocks
normal breathing, and that causes
blood oxygen levels to drop.
Normal blood oxygen levels above 94% can fall
below 90, 80, 70, 60, 50, 40, and even 30%.
This slow strangulation
forces the heart to overwork all night
to get oxygen to the brain.

* See *Death Knocks When The Lower Jaw Drops* on page 115

The Jaws & Dentures

Taking removable dentures out at night may be a killer. The tongue can be forced backwards into the throat and block the airway when the jaws do not have teeth or dentures to support them. If you have fewer than 24 teeth, or if you are missing a large number of back teeth, then wearing dentures at night may be healthier for you.

Removing dentures at night has been a standard practice for centuries and is still taught in dental schools.

Dentists have recommended nighttime denture removal for a number of reasons. Food gets trapped under dentures. Poor mouth cleaning habits can cause decay in remaining teeth. And early plastics used to make dentures had to be under water for some time to prevent cracking.

The standard practice of removing dentures at night must change. Today's newer plastics do not need to be in water to prevent fracture. People have access to better preventive dental care and mouth care instruction. The small amount of research in this area is very convincing.

Teeth and dentures support the jaws and maintain the oral gap—the tongue space between the upper and lower jaws. Sleeping infants and adults without teeth or dentures have nothing to keep the jaws apart, so the tongue can drop into the throat like a cork. This can cause sleep disorders.

A study published in September of 2000 found that removing complete dentures during sleep promoted respiratory disorders as well as increased the risk for both hypertension and cardiovascular disease. **This shows that taking dentures out when sleeping can be harmful.**[105]

**"Medicine is not only a science; it is also an art.
It does not consist of compounding
pills and plasters; it deals with the very processes
of life, which must be understood
before they may be guided."**

Theophrastus Bombast Von Hohenheim (1530) [106]

**"Nearly all men die of their medicines,
not of their diseases."**

J.B. Molier (1673) [107]

* **"Circling the world in the 1920s and 1930s,
Dr. Weston Price and his wife found the same
sinister pattern among 'primitive' populations...
Groups that followed their traditional
nature-based diets enjoyed good health and
vigor, and those that turned to the 'civilized' diet
or processed, sugar-laden foods soon developed a
variety of ills, including misshapen bones and
teeth—and the situation worsened
with each generation."**

Nutrition and Physical Degeneration—1939 [108]

See Dr. Weston Price's book *Nutrition and Physical
Degeneration* (pages 144 and 160)

The Jaws & Disease Prevention

Since the beginning of time man has searched for ways to prevent disease and live longer. The futile global search for "The Fountain of Youth" has unearthed some useful and some ridiculous things.

Chronic degenerative diseases continue in spite of man's best efforts. While many infectious diseases have been controlled by modern medicine, many chronic diseases such as cancer, diabetes, hypertension and heart disease persist. Hope remains for future cures.

Some see great promise in gene research, while others believe genes control only 25% of how healthy and how long we live. Cloned animals have major health problems. Even if a "perfect" human being could be cloned, cell mutations would likely cause disease.

Drugs, pharmaceutical medications or chemicals, manage some diseases but prevent very few. The many side effects of legal drugs have drawn recent attention.

Diet and airway have been somewhat ignored in research and clinical practice. While medicines command a high percentage of research dollars, diet and airway, two of the most important needs for human survival, have not. This must change. The human body needs good food and oxygen to be healthy and live long.

In 1939, Dr. Weston Price recorded decades of global research showing modern diet as a disease villain. His unique text and illustrations explain how diet affects the jaws and consequently the airway.

**Acute and chronic ear diseases
involve many factors,
and some are still unknown.**

**Many patients with inner ear dysfunction
suffer from dental disorders.**

**Patients with inner ear dysfunction, of unknown
cause, should have a dental exam.**

Dental treatment may improve ear symptoms.

HNO—1993 [109]

**Ear and jaw anatomy varies from person to
person. Some people have jaw joints which are
closer to the ear on one or both sides.**

**Some people have three body parts which differ in
location compared to other people.
(a nerve, a ligament and an artery)
One or all parts can pass through a small groove
in the skull called the petro-tympanic fissure and
physically connect the jaw joint to the ear.**

The Journal of Craniomandibular Practice—1995 [110]

**At times 30% of all annual prescriptions
distributed have been for ear disease.**

American Journal of Diseases of Children (1960)—1987 [111]

The Jaws & Ear Disease

Ear disease remains a puzzle for modern medicine, and is not readily preventable. In the U.S. alone, 10-15 million children suffer regularly from chronic ear infections, which are costly to manage. **Dental jaw treatment may help some people with ear problems.**

Some blame ear disease on genetics or random bad luck. Some say it is caused when one or both ears are exposed to loud sounds, different air, or different bacteria. Fact is, ear disease does not randomly pick people or ears. Some people never have ear trouble. Others have chronic problems in one or both ears. Something else is going on.

Progressive ear disease can involve one or both ears. Most often it occurs without the primary reason being known. It may start with unexplained chronic earwax build-up, a clogged ear feeling, or Eustachian tube dysfunction. It often gets worse with ear fluid build-up, then ringing in the ears (tinnitus), dizziness, vertigo, general loss of equilibrium, loss of hearing and eventually deafness.

Ear disease starts early in children. Statistically, one in three infants will not have ear "infections." Another one in three will have a few. The last one in three infants will suffer continuously with chronic ear problems, putting them at the highest risk for progressive ear disease throughout life.

Ear infection is the most frequent diagnosis made in physician offices for those under age 15. Since one third of all children are responsible for most of the repeat visits, any effective treatment would greatly reduce their suffering. Additionally, any truly effective treatment would greatly reduce the extremely high associated health care costs.

**Otitis media is currently
the most common diagnosis made by clinicians,
which has a major impact on managed care.**

Current Allergy Asthma Reports—2001 [112]

**The origin and cause of acute otitis media
and otitis media with effusion
is not yet understood.**

**The limited insight into the disease process
restricts rational and appropriate therapy.**

**Ear therapy is now based on pragmatic
responses; acute infection is treated with
antibiotics; persistent fluid is drained.**

**Further understanding of the pathogenesis of
middle-ear infection and its sequelae should yield
effective therapy.**

Pediatric Otolaryngology—1996 [113]

**Acute otitis media
is the most common disease for which
pediatricians prescribe antibiotics.**

Journal of Microbiology, Immunology and Infection—2001 [114]

Ear infection and otitis media are two terms used for decades to describe ear "infections" to parents. Both are usually treated the same way, with antibiotics. Otitis media is often called an infection, but it is better defined as inflammation of the middle ear. It currently represents a costly medical problem worldwide.

Diagnosis of otitis media in the U.S. increased from 9.1 million visits in 1975 to 24.5 million visits in 1990.[115] Related medical costs and lost wages in the U.S. alone amount to over $5 billion per year.[116] Otitis media is said to result from a bacterial or viral infection. Studies show this is not usually so. Global studies indicate as few as 25% of "infected" ears have disease-causing bacteria or viruses in them. So, up to 75% of the ears that seem infected are not.[117]

Otitis media ("ear infection") is a significant medical problem that deserves more research attention than it receives so significant costs and illness associated with it can be reduced.[118] In some cultures, otitis media related sickness is immense. Otitis media can be a factor in associated hearing loss, learning disabilities, and secondary central nervous system complications.

Prescription drugs have long been the routine treatment for otitis media and ear "infection." Since about one-third of all prescriptions distributed annually have been for ear disease, it is no surprise that roughly 7 million courses of antibiotics are used each year in the U.S. to treat ear conditions that do not require them.

The end of the 20th century brought some changes in the handling of ear disease. Scientists began to question the massive use of drugs as a primary ear treatment. Some antibiotics were found to have anti-inflammatory effects.[119] This may explain why some antibiotics appear to work in a few hours, when it would take many hours to kill bacteria.

**In 1998, physicians were so puzzled
as to why ears that appeared to be infected
actually tested sterile
that they began searching for "stealth
bacteria"—bacteria that purposely clump
together to hide from detection.**

The Philadelphia Inquirer—1998 [120]

**The future solution to otitis media,
acute or chronic,
does not lie in current therapy regimens.**

Otorhinolaryngology Head and Neck Surgery—1996 [121]

**Craniomandibular (jaw to skull) disorders are
frequently overlooked in the medical profession
as possible causes of hearing problems.**

The Functional Orthodontist—1995 [122]

In 1997, a New Zealand study of 2,089 otitis media patients showed no difference in treatment success rates between those treated with antibiotics and those not treated with antibiotics. [123]

In 1998, the scientific community expressed deep concerns to physicians about the excessive use of antibiotics. Bacteria were becoming more resistant to antibiotics. Children were becoming allergic from repeat exposures, putting them at lifelong risk for a number of reasons.

In 1998, the dangers of all prescription drugs drew even more attention. It was estimated that 100,000 people were dying each year from prescription drugs. At least 1 million people annually—one in four over a lifetime—were being hospitalized due to an adverse effect to a prescription drug. [124] Prescription drugs were said to kill more people each year than automobile and airplane accidents combined. [125]

Physicians were trapped between providing traditional care and using restraint with drugs. Even so, physicians continue to prescribe antibiotic drugs routinely to treat middle ear infections. [126] This form of ear disease "management" continues to this day.

The current medical approach offers little hope for any major breakthroughs in ear disease. The primary causes of ear infections remain unknown, so therapy is limited. Other aspects of progressive ear disease, such as ear wax, tubes, dizziness, vertigo, Meniere's, sudden hearing loss, and deafness of unknown origin all have similar problems with the current medical approach.

It is time for a new view and a new approach to ear disease prevention, diagnosis and treatment. Current treatment methods attempt to manage ear disease, but they can rarely prevent or cure it, nor predict who will have it.

*Children with deep dental overbites
are 2.8 times more likely to have ear tubes
(ear grommets) placed or recommended
by a pediatric otolaryngologist.

The Laryngoscope—2001 [127]

*The greatest cause of otitis media is an
over-closed or improper dental bite.
Otitis media can successfully be treated by using
primary molars (baby teeth).
A number of dental techniques can be used
to reshape the baby molars to open
a deep closed dental overbite.
This moves the lower jaw bone away from
the ears back at the jaw joints.

The Functional Orthodontist—1990 [128]

*After 20 ear problems in 2 ½ years,
I put plastic dental composites on my son's lower
back baby molar teeth to open the deep bite. His
lower jaw moved down and forward away from
his ears. He has not had ear problems since.

The Functional Orthodontist—1988 [129]

* See *Primary Molar Build-Up Brochure* (pages 144 and 160)

Veterinarians know what is going on with ear disease. They know that anatomy plays a big role. Different breeds of dogs with different ear and jaw anatomy have widely varying rates of ear infections.[130] While bacterial growth can cause inflammation, inflammation itself can be a main problem or it can be a breeding ground for bacterial growth.

In humans, just as in dogs, the anatomy of the ear and jaw largely determines whether ear problems occur. Humans differ in ear and jaw anatomy too. It can even vary greatly from one side to the other. This explains why some ears are affected and some are not. This also simply explains what current medical theories and views cannot.

Future breakthroughs in ear disease treatment will likely come from a dental jaw approach. It is the only sensible explanation for why one ear, both ears, or neither have chronic problems. It also easily explains why one person gets ear problems frequently and another does not. It even explains why problems run in families, where anatomy is similar.

Bacteria and viruses do not appear to be the primary causes of most false ear "infections" or true otitis media. Bacteria and viruses are secondary often and absent too often.

Pacifiers give a clue as to the real cause of many ear problems. Pacifier use, just like tooth grinding, can put constant pressure on jaw joints. Jaw joint inflammation leads to a warm moist environment where ear bacteria can grow or an ear can look red and feel inflamed, with no bacteria present.

Pacifier use doubles the risk of developing otitis media in infants under 12 months of age. Bottle-feeding increases the risk five times.[131] Pacifier use is responsible for at least 25% of otitis media attacks in children under age 3. [132] **Removing a pacifier from a child with chronic ear problems reduces likely future problems by about 50%.**

Acrylic resin bonded to the top surfaces of lower baby molars is an effective method to change the bite, and reduce or eliminate otitis media in young children between the ages of two to six years of age.

Journal of Clinical Pediatric Dentistry—1998 [133]

Patients with ear pain, dizziness, tinnitus, or ear fullness may have jaw-to-skull disorders. A dental bite plate placed to change the bite creates a new jaw-to-skull relationship and can significantly reduce ear symptoms.

Laryngoscope—1991 [134]

A person with less than 17 teeth has a 1.64 times greater chance of having hearing decline. Thereafter, every time a tooth is lost, a 4% hearing loss occurs.

Special Care in Dentistry—2001 [135]

Meniere's disease patients have a much higher incidence of jaw disorders.

Journal of Orofacial Pain—1996 [136]

Earwax is a sign a jaw is shifting out of balance toward one or both jaw joints. When the bite and the jaws are balanced, earwax tends to stop forming. Since dental doctors do not usually look in ears, and ear doctors do not usually look in mouths, this is not often seen. It is said that earwax knows when to show up to protect against bacteria and viruses, even to kill them. To the contrary, recent studies show many bacteria, viruses and fungi grow faster in earwax.

A new approach to ear disease prevention must start early while the jaws and jaw joints of the skull are forming. Tooth eruption and jaw growth need to be monitored regularly. Teething jaw forces do cause ear problems. Bite shifts and jaw shifts may benefit from corrective Functional Jaw Orthopedics as soon as possible. New ear disease diagnosis must include a look into the ears and mouth by someone with the knowledge and skill to see both sides of the problem. New ear treatments must include dental care at the earliest possible age, because dental treatment has been shown to effectively stop ear problems in some patients. New ear disease research needs to find out who can be helped by dental treatment and who cannot. Some ear damage is reversible and some is not.

If your child has chronic ear problems you may want to find a dentist skilled in Functional Jaw Orthopedics. If the bite is off in any of the three dimensions, the jaw can shift in a way that impacts the ears at the jaw joints. Studies show that balancing the bite and jaws may help. Children can have dental plastic composite bonded to baby teeth as early as age 2 to open an over closed dental bite and/or jaws.

If you are an adult with chronic ear problems such as ear pain, ear congestion, chronic ear disorder, dizziness, tinnitus, equilibrium problems, and sporadic hearing loss of unknown origin, consider consulting with an FJO dentist. People of all ages can have effective conservative jaw treatment to correct unbalanced bites or jaws. An added health benefit is that the ears often can get better too!

**Early orthodontic treatment
can be simpler, shorter and more favorable
than treating at a later age.**

**In children, dental cross bite
does not always cause facial lop-sidedness
or abnormal jaw movement.**

**However, if facial lop-sidedness is present
it will worsen during growth without
orthodontic treatment.**

The Bulletin of Tokyo Dental College—1995 [137]

**The first year of life
is the strongest period of jaw growth.**

**By age 6, about
90% of head growth and about
80% of jaw growth has already occurred.**

Facial Growth and Facial Orthopedics—1986 [138]

The Jaws & Early Orthodontics

Early orthodontic treatment is very controversial, even among dentists. Just the definition of early orthodontics can cause major conflicts of opinion. The advantages of early orthodontics should be better known because **braces at age 8 can be too late.**

Traditional orthodontics considers early treatment to be at age 8-9 years. This approach routinely suggests teeth are too big for a mouth. Often numerous baby teeth and adult teeth are then removed, on a regular basis, in a repeat tooth removal process called "serial extractions." Serial extractions cause dental arches to collapse, making small dental arches even smaller. This guided dental arch collapse is really active orthodontics and it works against jaw growth. In the 1970s, about 75% of patients had numerous baby teeth and/or 4 to 8 adult teeth removed for orthodontic treatment. These older approaches often result in reduced tongue and airway space.

Early Functional Jaw Orthopedics (FJO) appliance treatment can start at 2-6 years of age when indicated. The FJO approach works to increase dental arch size during early rapid growth periods, so it also supports breastfeeding for the first 6-12 months of life. Early FJO treatment has a philosophy opposite of traditional views. It works with jaw growth to increase tongue and airway space. When a mouth is too small, early action should be taken to increase space for the teeth and the tongue. By age 6 most jaw growth (80%) has occurred. Traditional orthodontics often waits to diagnose at age 7 and treat at age 8-12. Active FJO treatment at age 2-6 can more successfully influence tooth, jaw and airway growth.

If your child is 1-2 years of age, consider scheduling a first regular dental preventive visit soon. Then find an FJO dentist to examine the jaws and bite to be sure teeth and bones are developing and aligning well.

"The Lord prefers common-looking people.
That is the reason He makes so many of them."

Abraham Lincoln (1809-1865) [139]

**By 2 years of age to help prevent facial deformity
the mode of breathing should be assessed.**

**Obstruction of the nasal airway
is an important dysfunction.**

**To reduce jaw and facial abnormality,
better prenatal care, more breastfeeding,
and good nasal airway management
must occur to promote nasal breathing.**

The Angle Orthodontist—1979 [140]

**Orthopedic jaw appliances are able to change the
morphology and growth of the face.**

Facial Growth and Facial Orthopedics—1986 [141]

The Jaws & Faces

Faces differ greatly. Much of the difference is in how each of us looks in the lower half of the face. The shapes of our 3-dimensional jaws differ noticeably. They form the unique facial features seen below the eyes.

Some believe genetics pre-programs the face and cannot be easily changed. Others know that genetics is only one of many factors that affect facial growth.

Teeth and orthodontic techniques are two of the most important factors affecting jaw and facial growth.

Teeth are set in bone at birth like plant seeds in a pot. As teeth grow out of the bone into the mouth they help the bones of the jaws and face grow. When teeth are missing and not replaced, bone is lost and the jaws and face can be affected or deformed—during and/or after growth.

Orthodontic techniques vary greatly in how they influence jaw and facial growth. Proper jaw growth can be harmed by removing numerous teeth or by using backward forces. Proper facial growth can be helped by making room for crowded teeth with early phases of treatment and by using forward forces. You can see the difference between a narrow, pushed-back smile and a nice, broad, forward smile. You can also often see the difference in a face. Studies show the end smile result often depends upon the philosophy of the dentist providing the treatment and the techniques used.

If you want to change a face, Functional Jaw Orthopedics can start as early as age 2. Cooperative children can benefit from early orthodontic treatment. Traditional orthodontics at age 8-12 can be too late. Some adults can still benefit from FJO smile widening treatments. Adult treatments are more limited, may take more time, but have great benefits.

Headache and migraine sufferers lose more than 157 million workdays each year and industry loses 50 billion dollars per year."

National Headache Foundation—2002 [142]

Migraine and headache disorders generate a substantial disability burden and should be classified amongst major public health disorders. But, there remains a specific lack of public and professional awareness of the epidemiology of migraine and headache disorders and their impact on individual sufferers, their caregivers, family and colleagues, and on society itself.

World Health Organization—2000 [143]

Migraine disease is a serious health and disability problem. There is no known cure for the migraine disease, only treatments for the symptoms, which are not yet wholly effective.

Migraine Awareness Group—2002 [144]

Dental appliances have been found to reduce the number of migraine attacks by about 60%, especially in those who get frequent attacks.

British Dental Journal—1996 [145]

The Jaws & Headaches

About 45 million Americans suffer from chronic recurring headaches.[146] [147] The exact cause of migraine and other types of headache, even headache after trauma, is still unknown in many cases.[148] Medical therapy is often limited to treating symptoms with drugs. Dental jaw treatment helps some people with headaches and may do so without drugs or their side effects.

Medical treatment for headache historically has been by trial-and-error. One of the oldest recorded medical conditions 5000 years ago was headache. Old remedies such as drilling a hole in the skull had serious side-effects. Drugs used to treat headaches today have side effects too. Moreover, drugs do not generally treat related symptoms.

Dental treatment is often effective in reducing or eliminating headaches without drugs or surgery. It has been known for decades that headaches can be caused by dental or jaw problems. Toothache often causes facial pain, so fixing a dental problem can bring relief. Headache can cause or mimic a toothache. Some of these people get spontaneous relief without treatment, but they may have to wait months or years.

Hard and soft dental bite plates can often bring relief in days or weeks by balancing the dental bite. Bite and jaw imbalances often cause headaches. Sometimes just simple tooth adjustments can balance a bite and bring relief.

If you have chronic headaches, whether for just a few months or for many years, consider getting a medical and a dental FJO consult. Headache can be a symptom of a serious health problem such as a stroke or brain tumor. If you have chronic recurring headaches of unknown origin that have been evaluated by a physician, you may benefit from an FJO evaluation and FJO treatment, if indicated.

The known risk factors for coronary heart disease do not explain all of the clinical and epidemiological features of the disease. Dental health was significantly worse in patients with acute myocardial infarction.

British Medical Journal—1989 [149]

Dental disease persists as a major risk factor for heart disease even after adjusting for many lifestyle factors in the 13 known major risk factors.

Clinical Infectious Diseases—1995 [150]

Mean numbers of missing teeth were significantly higher among those who had a history of atherosclerotic vascular disease, heart failure, ischemic heart disease, and joint disease.

Special Care in Dentistry—1998 [151]

Twelve studies have associated dental conditions with either coronary heart disease or cerebral vascular accident. Because dental diseases are treatable, maintaining good oral health should receive the highest priority for a healthy life.

Compendium of Continuing Dental Education—2000 [152]

The Jaws & Heart Disease

Nearly 1 million Americans die from heart disease each year. It is the number one killer in the U.S. [153] Another 60 million Americans reportedly have some form of heart disease. Some primary causes of heart disease are still unknown. Widespread prevention is not possible and modern medicine is puzzled. Ignored teeth, jaws and airways are key pieces to the chronic heart disease puzzle.

Modern medicine can generally diagnose heart disease, but cannot routinely prevent it. Many people go undiagnosed as they have no signs or symptoms of disease. Even radiologists advertise full-body-scans to uncover the disease. In spite of this detection, prevention remains far-off.

Current theories on how to prevent heart disease seem to be failing. About half of those who die of heart disease die suddenly, without warning, in spite of swift emergency medical care. [154] Some people die without having known risk factors such as diabetes, hypertension, smoking, high cholesterol, triglycerides, socio-economic status, gender and age. People diet and exercise and still die prematurely.

Many theories or fads on how to prevent or reduce heart disease have surfaced over the past few decades. Theories run in cycles suggesting more or less butter, eggs, fat, meat, fruit, greens, alcohol, diet, sleep, stress, exercise, nuts, blood pressure and cholesterol drugs, etc. Even so, premature heart attacks kill those aged 30 to 60 rather often.

Recent studies show dental disease is a powerful independent risk factor for heart disease. Early evidence shows dental disease is a higher risk factor than smoking. One large study found those aged 25 to 49 with periodontal disease and/or no teeth had about a 72% higher risk of heart disease, and 2½ times the risk of death overall.

Tooth loss appears to be an independent predictor of abnormal electrocardiograph (ECG) heart findings in those over age 80, even after adjusting for other known risk factors.

Journal of Dental Research—2001 [155]

Complete tooth loss in young adults as opposed to older adults is associated with serious medical outcomes resulting in death.

Compendium of Continuing Dental Education—2000 [156]

Reduced chewing function has been linked to having fewer than 20 teeth present or to having removable dentures that fit poorly. Maintaining or re-establishing good chewing function is an integral part of the medical health care of frail or dependent elderly people.

Best Practice and Research Clinical Gastroenterology—2001 [157]

Tooth loss can be prevented through education, early diagnosis and regular dental care. Loss of all natural teeth can contribute to a person's psychological, social, and physical impairment.

Centers for Disease Control—2002 [158]

Some researchers suggest gum infection and/or gum inflammation causes heart damage.[159] [160] This gums-to-heart theory is weak.[161] The mouth and body are normally full of bacteria. Typically about billions of bacteria, 300 different types, are swallowed in saliva each day. Studies show heart disease grows in those with healthy gums and less bacteria.

The link between oral disease and heart disease can be better explained by tooth loss causing airway collapse, low night-time oxygen and then heart damage. When teeth are removed and not replaced, the jaws move closer together. Imagine standing under a tent when the support poles are removed. The space under the tent is reduced. If 6 to 10 back teeth are missing, the tongue and airway space is decreased. Dentists call this posterior bite collapse. Bite collapse in guinea pigs has been shown to harm the heart and body.[162]

Research in France and Hungary illustrates best the missing teeth-to-heart disease association. In France, men age 35-44 have an average of 27 teeth.[163] In Hungary, men age 35-44 average 20 teeth.[164] France has an "unexplained" low rate of heart disease, while Hungary's rate is quite high. [165] [166]

Worldwide statistics further support a connection between missing teeth and heart disease.[167] People of Japan, Canada, Spain, and France have few missing teeth at age 40, low rates of heart disease and long lifespan to about age 75. People of Brazil, Hungary and Poland have many missing teeth by age 40, high rates of heart disease and a short lifespan to age 58-69. The tooth-to-heart relation is globally clear.

If you want to live longer, try to save your teeth. It may save or extend your life. Researchers will debate how missing teeth cause heart disease for a while. Meanwhile, since a direct relationship exists, act now to save your teeth and replace missing teeth when possible. Other sections of this book should help you understand how tooth loss, airway collapse, hypoxia and human diseases relate.

"Man hath as many diseases
as a horse."

James Howell (1660) [168]

Horse TMJ can affect the whole horse.

Horse TMJ requires balancing the bite.

After TMJ treatment, it may take days for a horse
to get back to normal.

Horses get used to a new bite, and then begin to
feed properly again, regain lost weight, change
behaviors, and increase performance.

Horse owners commonly report that after TMJ
treatment, a horse not only listens better,
but also simply acts sweeter.

R Douglass CeqDT, Equine Dentist (2002) [169]

The Jaws & Horse TMJ, etc.

There are many names for temporo-mandibular jaw disorder (TMJ, TMD, CMD, etc.). Likewise there are many older views of TMJ which continue to say it is not a physical problem. A look at horse TMJ may help to show how human TMJ disorders do exist physically.

Some say TMJ is mostly psychological. They cling to stale beliefs and use drugs as a main treatment. They show bias by criticizing clinicians who document successful jaw therapy results.[170] **The truth is, TMJ is a physical problem.**

Horses get TMJ disorders just like humans! [171] Horse TMJ occurs when horse teeth, which wear faster than human teeth, wear unevenly. Abnormal tooth wear can cause the bite to shift. Then the jaws shift. When horse jaws shift they can put pressure on one or both jaw joints. That is when the horse begins to suffer, and the suffering shows.

Horse TMJ can affect the whole horse. Equine dentists, veterinarians and horse handler professionals see major behavioral changes. Horses with TMJ tend to drop feed, lose weight, head-tilt, change gait, react differently to the bit, misbehave and go through visible attitude changes.[172]

When horse TMJ is diagnosed, balancing the bite, called floating, is the effective therapy.[173] Horse teeth grow and wear continuously. So horses need routine exams and adjustments for teeth, jaws and TMJs that are out of balance. Just like horses, humans respond to bite and jaw balancing. Treatments differ because human teeth do not keep growing.

If you have TMJ problems, you may want to find an FJO dentist who knows about teeth and jaws. If we put horse sense into our view of human TMJ, fewer drugs would be used, and we could save lots of time, money and pain.

In a sleep study
of 31 young hypertensive men,
all of them had indirect signs of obstructive sleep
apnea, as compared with controls.
The study concluded the trigger for arterial
hypertension to be the lungs, due to sub-clinical
obstruction of the upper airways.

Terapevticheskii Arkhiv—2001 [174]

The search for the primary cause
of hypertension has occurred during the day,
but the killer works mostly at night.
During sleep, choking them hundreds of times in
a night, gravity pulls the lower jaw, tongue,
uvula and other tissues into the throat.
The real villain, a blocked airway, can be heard
in the unique choking sounds of
snores, groans, grunts, and gasps.

Early diagnosis and treatment
of sleep-related breathing disorders may
make patients feel much better, (something
anti-hypertensive drugs do not always do), and
may reduce blood pressure and prevent the
progression of renal (kidney) and cardiovascular
(heart) damage as well.

Nephrology Dialysis Transplantation—1997 [175]

The Jaws & Hypertension

Hypertension, known as high blood pressure, continues to be a leading cause of death. Most hypertension occurs for unknown reasons, and it is usually progressive. Therapy is generally limited to drugs. **Dental jaw treatment can help with this problem and may one day be a chief means of therapy and prevention.**

Primary hypertension or essential hypertension is high blood pressure of unknown origin. 95% of those with high blood pressure have primary hypertension. The other 5% have rare secondary or identifiable hypertension. Secondary hypertension has a recognized cause such as renal disease.[176]

High blood pressure can be documented and somewhat controlled by modern medicine, but it cannot be routinely prevented. The common disease process often progresses to kidney and heart disease, followed by death. Nephrologists, kidney physicians, know this process and the importance of finding the true causes of hypertension.

Blood oxygen dipping during sleep is a main cause of hypertension and morning heart attack. Nighttime low oxygen (hypoxia) changes circadian rhythms and affects both blood and blood pressures during the day. Measuring high blood pressure during daytime does not address night causes.

If you have hypertension, you may want to seek out rare nighttime pulse-oximetry oxygen screening. A small portable memory pulse-oximeter attached to your finger records several nights of sleep data in your own bed. A sleep medicine physician can then review oxygen level results and recommend treatment, if appropriate. **If FJO dental devices are used to bring the jaw forward and open the airway, the effectiveness can be checked by pulse-oximetry.**

Sleep-related breathing disorders
ranging from habitual snoring to airway
resistance and airway obstruction, along with
obstructive sleep apnea syndrome (OSAS),
are now recognized as major health problems.

The American Journal of Medicine—2000 [177]

Sleep Disorder is an independent risk factor for:
Auto Accident
Brain Damage
Daytime Sleepiness
Diabetes
Heart Attack
Heart Disease
Hypertension
Kidney Disease
Morning Heart Attack
Premature Death
Stroke

Oral dental appliances that position the lower jaw
forward during sleep and open the airway
are valuable sleep disorder treatment alternatives
to CPAP (a machine that pumps air into the lungs
through a mask) and surgery.

Therapeutische Umschau. Revue Therapeutique—2000 [178]

The Jaws & Sleep Disorders

S leep disorders are slowly being recognized as major factors in human illness and premature death. Although sleep apnea and sleep disordered breathing are increasingly making the news, modern medical screening and treatment are not reaching the majority of people at risk. **Dental jaw treatment can help some people with this problem.**

Sleep disorders affect 5-20% or more of the population and are a burden to modern society. Over 30 million people snore. Millions suffer from sleep disorders which can lead to high blood pressure, heart disease and even early death. More than 90% of these people go undiagnosed and untreated. Most people with sleep disorders do not know it, but the people they live and sleep with often do. Spouse and companionship difficulties, poor job performance, lost productivity, social problems, mood swings, morning headaches, depression, and sleepiness can result. Sleep disorders are blamed for $16 billion per year in direct medical costs and $56 billion per year in sleep-related automobile accidents. Patients with sleep apnea are 2 to 7 times more likely to cause an automobile accident.[179] [180] This is a health tragedy.

Obstructive sleep apnea, a form of sleep disorder, starts when blocked airways cause low levels of blood oxygen, known as hypoxia. Hypoxia interrupts breathing patterns (apnea) and results in a broad range of chronic illnesses, full body changes and sometimes sudden death.

If you live near a fire station, the morning fire alarms you hear between 4 A.M. and 9 A.M. may not be for fires.[181] Sleep disordered breathing often causes morning heart attack. The dead or dying victim is usually found one step out of bed or sitting on the toilet—the two common places to die from problems that may involve sleep disorders. [182]

Epworth Sleepiness Scale

The Epworth Sleepiness Scale is a short quiz designed to help screen whether you have a sleep disorder. Rate from 0 to 3 your chance of dozing in the eight listed situations. Add the eight ratings to get a **Total Epworth Sleepiness Score.**

Rating Guide:

Would never dose	=> 0
Slight chance of dozing	=> 1
Moderated chance of dozing	=> 2
High chance of dozing	=> 3

Situation:	Chance of Dozing:
1. Sitting and reading	_____
2. Watching TV	_____
3. Sitting, inactive in public	_____
4. Car passenger (for an hour)	_____
5. Lying down in the afternoon	_____
6. Sitting and talking to someone	_____
7. Sitting quietly after lunch (no alcohol)	_____
8. Stopped for a few minutes in traffic	_____

Total Epworth Sleepiness Score: _____

A total score of 10 or more suggests you may need further evaluation to determine if you have a sleep disorder and/or sleep disordered breathing. If you think you have sleep apnea, discuss it with a medical or dental doctor familiar with sleep disorders. **You can even consult directly with a sleep medicine physician. Do not postpone needed treatment!**

Sleep medicine physicians currently use overnight sleep studies to diagnose sleep disorders. They often prescribe Continuous Positive Air Pressure (CPAP) pumps to force air into the lungs. CPAP is considered the "gold standard" for treating sleep disorders. Since a facemask must be worn all night long, and the pump is noisy, many people do not wear it long term, so the disorder continues.

Ear Nose and Throat physicians offer a variety of surgeries to reduce sleep disorders: nasal surgery, uvula and throat tissue removal surgery or tissue shrinkage. Studies give mixed reviews of these treatment costs vs. their benefits. Considering surgery is rather irreversible, it makes sense to also learn about all non-surgical treatment options.

Dental devices worn at night are a major non-surgical treatment option for snoring, sleep apnea and certain other sleep disorders. Recent research shows that oral dental devices can be effective for mild, moderate and even severe sleep apnea, in some cases.[183]

Oral device designs vary but basically aim to keep the airway open during sleep. They keep the lower jaw forward, opening the throat airway space, like the jaw-thrust first step in CPR. The best mouth appliance designs hold onto the teeth, do not move the teeth, and do not over stress or pain the jaw joints when worn nightly. Oral devices and the patients wearing them should be routinely examined as they can cause jaws to grow in children and teenagers.

FJO dentists are in a prime position to help screen for and treat people with sleep disorders. Dentists could screen for sleep disorders at dental visits using questionnaires and even provide overnight pulse-oximetry data gathering screening services. They could then coordinate diagnosis, treatment planning and actual therapy with sleep physicians. **Dental devices can help keep the airway open during sleep, even in patients with severe sleep disorder.**[184]

**The American Academy of Pediatrics
issued new guidelines in 2002 in an attempt to
diagnose and manage children with obstructive
sleep apnea syndrome (OSAS).**

**All children are to be screened for snoring.
For those diagnosed with OSAS, adenoid and
tonsil removal is to be the first treatment.**

Pediatrics—2002 [185]

**In Korea, as in other parts of the world,
the frequency of hypertension was found to be
higher in snorers compared to non-snorers.**

The Korean Journal of Internal Medicine—2001 [186]

**Habitual snoring is deadly and a main symptom
of sleep apnea syndrome (SAS), which
occurs in 4 to 7% of adults.
Patients with SAS who go without treatment,
have about a 37% increased chance
of being dead within 8 years.**

Anales De Medicina Interna—1999 [187]

The Jaws & Snoring

S noring is often a cry for help, not just an embarrassing sound. Modern medicine practically ignored this nighttime distress signal until recently. Snoring is gaining ground as an independent sign of sleep disordered breathing, and both should be taken seriously. **FJO dentists can help screen for snorers and help provide snore treatment.**

Snoring is a clear signal that an airway is blocked. Enlarged tonsils and adenoids easily block airways in children and in some adults. An undergrown small jaw can result in a small airway that is more easily blocked when a sleeping jaw drops. Compressed and crowded throat tissues can result in choking a sleeper hundreds of times a night.

Habitual snoring often signals the presence of dangerous nighttime sleep disorders. Sleep disorders are now known to be an independent risk factor for a number of diseases, including hypertension, cardiovascular disease, cerebrovascular disease (stroke) [188] and diabetic insulin resistance. [189]

Snoring alone is hard on the heart and brain. Research suggests that snorers have low night oxygen even if they do not have a sleep disorder.[190] Snoring has been found to be a predictor of poor school performance. A study that compared childhood snoring at 2 to 6 years of age to school performance at 13 to 14 years of age found children with lower performance in middle school were more likely to have snored during early childhood. They were also more likely to require later tonsil and adenoid removal.[191]

If you snore, tell your doctors. Sleep medicine physicians can determine if you have sleep disordered breathing and review treatment options (tonsil removal, oral device or CPAP). **FJO dentists can design mouthpieces to open your airway and reduce snoring or sleep disordered breathing.**

Enlarged tonsils and adenoids can cause major health problems. Symptoms may disappear after tonsil and adenoid removal.

Laryngologie, Rhinologie, Otologie—1978 [192]

Hypertrophy (enlargement) of the tonsils and adenoids is the most common cause of obstructive sleep apnea in children.

International Journal Pediatric Otorhinolaryngology—1987 [193]

Infants with upper airway obstruction, caused by adenotonsillar hypertrophy, often suffer from sudden death.

Nippon Jibiinkoka Gakkai Kaiho—1999 [194]

Tonsil removal may improve school performance.

Pediatrics—1998 [195]

Presence of dental cross bite was high in children with severe airway obstruction, particularly in those with hypertrophied adenoids and tonsils.

The Journal of Clinical Pediatric Dentistry—1994 [196]

The Jaws & Tonsils

Enlarged tonsils or adenoids can block the airway and breathing, and even be life threatening.[197] The tonsils on both sides of the throat, and the adenoids located above the throat are clumps of specialized immune system tissues. Tonsils can act like sponges for bacteria. [198] Surface throat swabs can be fairly unreliable and invalid.[199] **Snoring** may signal a tonsil-blocked (obstructed) airway.

About forty years ago it was routine to remove tonsils and adenoids in children. This does not happen today for a number of reasons including surgical risk, insurance issues, law suit issues, and the controversial belief that they are important for a good immune system.[200 201]

Enlarged tonsils and adenoids can cause chronic airway obstruction and chronic health problems such as bad breath, frequent illness, snoring, bad swallow habits, breathing problems, crooked teeth and jaws, facial deformity, fatigue, sleep disorder, sleep apnea, poor health, high blood pressure, right-side-heart enlargement (cor pulmonale), slow growth, unseen heart damage, heart failure and death.[202 203]

Tonsil and adenoid removal (adenotonsillectomy) can often reverse the signs and symptoms related to a blocked airway. If removal is indicated, consider removing both tonsils and adenoids at one time. If only one set of tissues is removed, it is often necessary to remove the other at a later date. Surgical removal has risks and can be painful, but better overall health may be a long term benefit.

If you or your child have enlarged tonsils or adenoids, ask your doctor if they should be removed. Patients with airway obstruction should be screened for already-present heart damage before tonsil or adenoid removal so special treatment precautions can be taken. [204]

The August 2000 Surgeon General's report
confirmed that neglected, vulnerable populations
in the United States are not adequately receiving
oral health services.

Dental Clinics of North America—2001 [205]

A study of mentally retarded children found
oral hygiene and periodontal health were poor
and most children had gingival bleeding.

Community Dental Oral Epidemiology—1985 [206]

Early orthodontic treatment
of children with Down's syndrome can lessen or
even normalize severe tongue protrusion and
mouth closure dysfunctions.

Journal of Orofacial Orthopedics— 2001 [207]

Patients with Down's syndrome should
be screened for sleep apnea.

American Family Physician—2001 [208]

Oral appliances are useful as an alternative to
relieve sleep apnea in patients with mental
deficiencies and neuromuscular disabilities such
as Cerebral Palsy and Down syndrome.

Journal of Prosthetic Dentistry—1999 [209]

The Jaws & The Forgotten

The teeth and jaws of those with disabilities are often considered a low priority and somewhat ignored.[210] The forgotten—the disabled, the elderly, and the institutionalized—like everyone else, need teeth to support their jaws, which then can support their airway.

The forgotten have a hard time getting routine dental care. Many of these patients lack transportation, money, and even the simple ability to travel to a dental office for treatment. Few hospitals and institutions are staffed or equipped to provide specialized dental care. Few dentists are trained or equipped to provide out-patient sedation, which is needed by some patients with disabilities. All important preventive dental care is rarely a main concern of most policy makers.

Some of these children and adults go for years without dental treatment. Specialized care requires dentists to charge much higher fees to those least able to afford it. While government programs help the disabled, the elderly and the institutionalized in many ways, dental care is generally not covered. In some states, Medicaid does not cover dental care for adults with Cerebral Palsy or Down's syndrome.

Assisting the disabled financially to have greater access to quality dental care will help them health-wise. There is clear evidence that loss of teeth worsens health. Those with disabilities living in institutions lose their teeth, get sicker, and die sooner than those living in family homes. This may be a key reason why those with Down's syndrome recently doubled their life span as more now live at home.

If you want to help those who need help the most, contact your politicians. Advise them of your concerns. Ask them to take action to help those with disabilities to receive needed dental care, especially preventive dental care.

From the first day, all through life, the jaws help maintain the vital human airway.

Essentials of Facial Growth—1996 [211]

The biting forces of chewing measure about 95 pounds at the front incisor teeth, 218 pounds at the middle bicuspid teeth, and 266 pounds at the back molar teeth.

United University of Sichuan—1994 [212]

Temporomandibular Joint Syndrome (TMJ): "It nearly ruined my life. It's an incredibly painful condition. I couldn't chew, I had severe headaches and muscle spasm in my face, neck and back. I lost my job and nearly lost my husband. For two years the doctors didn't know what was wrong with me. I was suicidal because of the pain and was even sent to a mental health facility! As far as not being able to sleep with an appliance in the mouth, consider the alternatives: three operations, $250,000 in medical bills and six years in hell!"

The Baltimore Sun Paper—1988 [213]

Functional Jaw Orthopedics

Paraphrased Article Reprint Permission Granted by the AAFO
The Functional Orthodontist—Spring 2001

Functional Jaw Orthopedics (FJO) is the newest, most progressive form of orthodontics. FJO dentists will lead dentistry and medicine into a new world of medical dentistry. Patients will have new options for effective alternative treatment.[214]

Chewing puts 95 to 266 pounds of biting force on teeth. These forces of chewing, along with grinding, clenching, and swallowing habits, all contribute to lifelong changes in teeth, bone and tissues. Normal aging and dental treatment can affect tooth position and jaw position throughout life. These changes can be for better or for worse.

Heavy biting forces are transferred to the jaw joints during chewing and also to a smaller degree during clenching, grinding or swallowing. A space between the back ends of the lower jawbone and the bone of the joints along with a special joint cartilage usually provide protection. Jaws and jaw joints are usually very resilient, especially when protected by balanced tooth support.

Simple tooth imbalances, which force the lower jaw to shift, can cause jaw, jaw joint, head and body damage. If a jaw shifts toward one or both joints, biting forces transferred to the jaw joints can then lead to jawbone and joint degeneration. This can frequently be seen on radiographs. Jaw joint degeneration is a principal cause or principal result of both facial bone changes and unstable occlusion (bites) in patients with a full set of teeth. [215]

Enough stress and strain can cause jaw and jaw joint dysfunction (TMJ), which is hard to diagnose and treat. **That is why TMJ disorder is called "The Great Imposter."**

**Teeth hit like cogs in a wheel, so when teeth are
moved the lower jaw can be repositioned.
The lower jaw can then strain the many muscles,
ligaments, vessels nerves, bones and two jaw
joints to which it is attached.
The forces of chewing, age changes and many
dental treatments can affect tooth position and
jaw position for better or for worse.**

The Functional Orthodontist—1988 [216]

**Functional Jaw Orthopedic appliances
can result in "a significant increase in lower
jaw growth and development."**

The Functional Orthodontist—1997 [217]

**To provide efficient orthodontic and
orthopedic treatment...to obtain esthetic
and functional jaw corrections...
four essential rules must be taken care of:
finding the best therapeutic choice,
choosing the best moment to start treatment,
initiating an efficient unlocking (of the jaw)
and providing an overall treatment.**

L' Orthodontie Francaise—2000 [218]

Dentists (Doctors of Dentistry) spend a lifetime saving, repairing, and replacing teeth for patients over their lifetime.

Dental specialists in tooth movement (orthodontists) move teeth in people on average starting at 12 years of age. More patients are starting as early as age 8, but most are not.

Functional Jaw Orthopedics involves changing the relationships of teeth, bone, muscles and tissues of the upper and lower jaws, jaw joints and skull. Dentists who provide FJO treatment do not just move teeth. FJO dentists need extensive knowledge, skills, and experience, in order to provide the broad range of unique FJO treatments. Some FJO treatments have medical effects.

New FJO dentists, including general dentists, pedodontists (children's dentist) and orthodontists treat crooked teeth and jaws at earlier ages, some as early as age 2. Jaw growth is vital between birth and age 8, so a great gap in healthcare exists. FJO dentists are filling this healthcare void.

The FJO approach treats teeth and jaws starting at birth. The purpose is to manage growth, development and deformation. With this method, dental techniques are used in one or more phases of treatment to design beautiful, broad, healthy smiles and give good dental function when possible.

Traditional orthodontics performed around age 12 provides treatment after most of the jaw growth has already occurred. Even braces at age 8 can be too late. While orthodontic treatments are constantly evolving, few theories advocate continuous monitoring of the jaws throughout life. A dental tooth and gum exam is not the same as a jaw exam.

The FJO philosophy is that jaw formation should be checked at an earlier age, even at birth. Today jaws are evaluated at too late an age, after most jaw growth occurs.

**Health professionals
should inform expectant mothers
about the dental and facial advantages
of breastfeeding.**

ASDC Journal of Dentistry for Children—1996 [219]

**Pacifier use was found to be associated with
shorter duration of breastfeeding.**

Acta Paediatrica—1999 [220]

**Soy formula contains large amounts of
phyto-estrogen isoflavones which can act like
estrogen, while breastmilk has negligible
amounts of isoflavones.**

Lancet—1997 [221]

**It has been found that the frequency of feedings
with soy-based milk formulas in early life was
significantly higher in children with
autoimmune thyroid disease.**

Journal of the American College of Nutrition—1990 [222]

Jaws form and deform slowly with age. Periodic jaw check-ups should occur as often as dental check-ups. Short phases of treatment should be advised when appropriate to guide jaw growth and development and then to safeguard it.

FJO planning should begin with parental counseling long before a baby is born. Maternal health at conception can severely impact jaw formation and deformation. Maternal diet, drug and alcohol habits can also severely affect fetal growth and development. Vitamin deficiencies are directly related to fetal bone deformation.

Fetal alcohol syndrome is a major cause of fetal mal-formation. Mothers-to-be should be encouraged to follow advice from their healthcare providers regarding topics ranging from proper nutrition to use of drugs. Fathers-to-be should be educated to understand the extensive health and financial benefits of good parental health prior to conception.

Fetal exposures that result in the worst infant abnormalities are not well understood. [223] [224] When it comes to the palate there is clear evidence that certain fetal exposures, especially in the first trimester, result in high, narrow palates and cleft palates. Basic vitamin deficiencies or steroid use can also interfere with proper bone growth.

Some infant formulas contain soy which is a potent imitator of estrogen. Estrogen mimickers are suspected of causing numerous abnormalities by their hormonal and non-hormonal effects.[225] Research has shown that daily exposure of infants to the bioactive isoflavones in soy infant-formulas is 6-11 times higher on a body weight basis than the dose necessary to cause hormonal effects in adults consuming soy foods.[226] The implications of such excessive exposure to endocrine-disrupting agents during fetal and infant development are grave. **Exclusive breast-feeding has been found to reduce this potentially dangerous exposure while aiding proper jaw and airway development.**

Unexplained deaths from intrauterine hypoxia (low oxygen) occur in about 1 in 1,000 pregnancies near term. Over 90% of these dead infants are about normal size.

The Australian & New Zealand
Journal of Obstetrics & Gynaecology—1986 [227]

Pregnancy can be complicated by obstructive sleep apnea, which may produce hypoxia, sleep disruption and potential adverse effects on the mother and fetus, including pre-eclampsia and low birth weight.

Obstetrical & Gynecological Survey—1996 [228]

The true incidence of sleep disordered breathing during pregnancy remains unknown.
Given the possible consequences of sleep apnea for fetal outcome, any significant sleep-disordered breathing is probably an indication for treatment.

Clinics in Chest Medicine—1992 [229]

Dentists have used oral appliances for decades to treat snoring and obstructive sleep apnea.

Otolaryngol and Head and Neck Surgery—2000 [230]

Hypoxia, lack of oxygen, is well known to cause fetal and infant abnormalities, growth retardation, and death. Hypoxia should be a major concern during pregnancy, especially in the third trimester, when snoring and sleep apnea increase. Snoring, common in pregnancy, is a sign of pregnancy-induced hypertension. Snoring signals a risk of fetal growth retardation.[231]

At the present time, pregnant mothers are not routinely screened for nighttime apnea related low oxygen. [232] Hypoxic pregnant women should be prescribed simple effective ways to increase their reduced oxygen levels, like the use of nasal strips or oral devices. Routine sleep apnea and/or low oxygen screening for pregnant women does not occur today but it should become routine in the future. Dentists must become directly involved in lifesaving airway maintenance and expansion, especially in pregnant women. This concept is extremely important during each trimester of pregnancy.

FJO strategies should be implemented at birth to manage the orthopedic forces placed on the jaws of the infant during labor and delivery. Just like forces of delivery can create a cone-headed child, they can also severely distort the maxilla and mandible. We are in the early stages of understanding the long-term impact of different delivery methods. It is not current protocol to have special craniosacral (jaw-skull-spine) evaluation of infants at birth. I believe it will be in the future. Likewise, newborn palate and nasal septum manipulation to correct deformed palates at birth will be refined and administered more in the future.[233] Parents-to-be should be encouraged to discuss birthing plans with their birth care providers as early as possible.

Exclusive breast-feeding is early FJO treatment and should be strongly recommended for about 6 months.[234] Recently released U.S. Surgeon General guidelines call for at least one year of breastfeeding.[235]

Breastfeeding during the first 6 months has a protective effect against respiratory and gastrointestinal illness, and all illnesses.

Journal of Paediatrics and Child Health—1995 [236]

Breastfeeding is protective against atopic disease including atopic eczema, food allergy, and respiratory allergy—throughout childhood and adolescence.

Lancet—1995 [237]

Breastfeeding rates in the U.S. hit an all time low in 1973 with 26% of new mothers choosing it as the method to use. The baby-boomer population, whose current ages are between 29 and 50 years, now make up 40% of the adult population, with an estimated 75 million adults in the U.S.... ....this has resulted in a lack of available and/or knowledgeable female relatives to provide breastfeeding guidance.

The Support of Breastfeeding—1998 [238]

Breastfeeding places beneficial orthopedic forces on the jaws, similar to the forces of Functional Jaw Orthopedics.

The Functional Orthodontist—2001 [239]

Studies show that about six months of exclusive breast-feeding dramatically reduces a number of major chronic infant illnesses.[240] Although this advice goes against modern cultural trends, infant feeding choices and related acquired habits all affect jaw development and deformation.

Exclusive breast-feeding saves a phenomenal amount of time, money and pain. Use of artificial breast milk (infant formula) is associated with higher rates of infection, pneumonia, gastroenteritis, allergies, asthma, SIDS, lymphoma, obesity, heart disease, ulcerative colitis and Crohn's disease, as well as lower intelligence scores and school performance. World Health Organization policy restricts the marketing of artificial breast milk to pregnant women because of the severe consequences to infants.[241]

New parents need to see the benefits of exclusive breast-feeding to understand the need to plan about 6 months of exclusive breast-feeding. Once they see how jaws grow differently with breast suckling than with infant bottle sucking, they will most likely consider breastfeeding a priority and find it important to consult with a certified breast-feeding consultant months before delivery.

The orthopedic forces of infant feeding act on the jaws during the strongest postnatal growth period—the first year.[242] While the benefits of breast milk over formula are well known and documented, the positive orthopedic jaw effects of breast suckling are not. Breast suckling forces on the jaws are opposite the forces of bottle or pacifier sucking.

Forward forces of breast suckling act to expand dental arches and jaws—like FJO appliances. Suckling forces develop palatal arches in the anterior and posterior regions. Suckling forces follow normal developmental growth directions of the maxilla and mandible, allowing both to reach their genetic potentials. Suckling forces differ dramatically from the arch-constricting effects of sucking.

**Functional repeat forward jaw motion
(action similar to breast suckling)
(action opposite of bottle or pacifier sucking)
appears to be the best way to promote
proper lower jaw growth and lengthening.**

*Maxillofacial Orthopedics:
A Clinical Approach for the Growing Child—1984* [243]

Pacifiers interfere with breastfeeding.

Pediatrics—1999 [244]

**Women who breastfeed and their infants
have lower health care costs compared with
those who formula feed.**

Birth—2002 [245]

**Cesarean section is a persistent and significant
barrier to beginning early breastfeeding.**

Birth—2002 [246]

**Breastfeeding benefits the mother too.
It reduces the risk of postpartum blood loss,
lowers the risk of pre-menopausal breast cancer
and also reduces the risk of ovarian cancer.**

Clinics in Perinatology—1999 [247]

Backward forces of bottle and pacifier sucking constrict dental arches and jaws, dramatically increasing malocclusions. [248] [249] Sucking forces constrict palatal arches, especially in the anterior canine regions. The forces of sucking oppose normal developmental growth directions of both the maxilla and mandible, preventing them from reaching their genetic potential. Narrowed maxillary arches additionally interfere with and prevent normal mandibular arch, jaw growth and forward positioning. The longer and stronger an infant sucks, the more damage is done. [250]

Twenty-five years of research comparing ancient skulls to modern day skulls has confirmed a dramatic reduction in size of the jaws in modern times. [251] Anthropologists blame soft diets for shrinking human jaw size compared to ancient jaws. In fact, nutrient content of the diet and mechanical actions of infant feeding better explain the large differences. [252]

Exceptions to patterns of jaw development do exist. So it should be understood that factors that cause and prevent malocclusion are not universal; they are strictly more-than-likely to happen. Some bottle-fed children have perfect occlusions, and some breast-fed infants have horrid ones. Forces on jaws are multi-factorial and variable.

Studies are increasingly concluding the method of infant feeding (suckling vs. sucking) has lifelong health consequences. It makes sense that feeding forces impact jaw structures that surround the human airway (the gateway-to-the-human-airway) and join to the skull. The literature is clear: Breast suckling for about 6 months decreases malocclusion, promotes nasal breathing and gives an infant dozens of health advantages over a lifetime. The literature is also clear. Bottle sucking and particularly pacifier sucking promote malocclusion, mouth breathing and infant illness.

Early orthodontic treatment is effective and desirable in specific situations.

Journal of the American Dental Association—2000 [253]

Early orthodontic treatment can be simpler, shorter and more favorable than treating at a later age. In children, dental cross bite does not always cause facial lop-sidedness or abnormal jaw movement. However, if facial lop-sidedness is present it will worsen during growth without orthodontic treatment.

The Bulletin of Tokyo Dental College—1995 [254]

The important benefits of early treatment should not be denied because of concerns that a few may still require further treatment later.

The Angle Orthodontist—1983 [255]

For deep bites, early orthodontics should start before all baby teeth fall out in order to allow the lower jaw to move forward with normal growth.

Australian Orthodontic Journal—2001 [256]

When a dental malocclusion exists, the time to make major non-surgical corrections is limited. By age six, the upper and lower jaw structures have reached about 80% of their full growth. As the maxilla and mandible grow, regular jaw exams with appropriate interceptive FJO treatment phases guide jaw growth with potential for incredible results.

Early FJO treatment can be revolutionary early interception and medical dentistry prevention. A dental malocclusion can appear innocent, but it can still cause facial lopsidedness in the absence of orthodontic treatment.[257] It is better to work early and progressively in phases, as a child grows and develops, rather than to limit treatment options at a much later age and later stage of development.

Early FJO philosophies differ considerably from traditional orthodontics. The age when active treatment starts is but one example. Traditional orthodontic diagnosis is recommended by age 7 and active appliance treatment on average begins at age 12. The FJO approach encourages much earlier diagnosis and treatment with arch and vertical development starting as early as age 2 or 3. The benefits of early diagnosis and treatment are easily recognized. The fact is orthodontic treatment at age 8 can be much too late. [258]

FJO treatments and traditional orthodontic treatments also differ profoundly on how to handle early tooth crowding problems. Traditional treatments often involve prescribing the lengthy repeat process of serial tooth extraction.[259] This invasive and costly sequential tooth removal process causes loss of tooth space and airway space as dental arches collapse. FJO techniques act in a totally opposite fashion to actively guide dental arch development in order to make room for erupting teeth. Since FJO-guided arch development can also enhance jaw growth, the benefits are readily visible. A further benefit is that FJO treatment guides the lower jaw forward to help enlarge the airway.

"Every tooth in a man's head
is more valuable to him than a diamond."

Cervantes: Don Quixote—1605 [260]

Smokers have both more frequent and more
severe periodontal disease, as well as higher
incidence of tooth loss and total tooth loss,
compared to non-smokers.

Annals of Periodontology—1998 [261]

"About 50% of periodontal disease in young
adults is attributable to cigarette smoking."

Gesundheitswesen—2000 [262]

A study of men from age 70 to 79 found
that a decline in dental condition and dental
function was significantly associated with a lower
capacity in brain function, vision, hearing,
lung volume, heart volume, muscle strength
and bone mineral content.
In addition, the 70 year olds that lived to age 79
had better dental condition than those who died.

Community Dental Oral Epidemiology—1990 [263]

FJO treatments utilize a broad range of appliances and techniques. This allows each patient to be treated individually, instead of being fit into some narrow time line or treatment method. Removable appliances place orthodontic and orthopedic forces on teeth and jaws. They can be made of metal, plastic or both and can be used beginning at age three. Fixed appliances can be metal, plastic, ceramic or combination thereof.

A unique FJO skill, "braces-without-braces," uses dental composite bonding materials to move teeth and reposition jaws. It can even be used before age two. Bonding, appliances, single lower anterior tooth removal and 2nd molar replacement are all FJO tools. FJO theory is pioneering the use of dental appliances (mandibular advancing positioners — MAPs) for snoring and sleep apnea.

There are dozens of great reasons for patients to choose FJO treatment. FJO treatment can help develop more attractive faces and smiles and open airways. Early FJO treatment corrects small problems before they grow bigger, leading to fewer "serial" extractions and fewer overall extractions. Adults of all ages can be treated with FJO therapy, which helps develop healthier jaws, TM joints and balanced bites. FJO treatment can even prevent surgery.

Providing FJO treatment is rewarding because it can be powerful, effective medical dentistry. FJO therapy can help to improve a patient's self image and also provide positive lifelong effects. It promotes good dental function, which has multiple medical benefits.

Studies show that good dental function is significantly associated with better cognitive thought, better vision, better hearing, better lung volume, better heart volume, greater muscle strength, better bone mineral content, fewer heart attacks and a longer life.[264][265]

**Functional Jaw Orthopedic (FJO) treatment
will be a healing art of the future
for some conditions.**

**Few other forms of treatment
can approach the broad, swift, lasting results
achieved by FJO treatment,
whether surgical, non-surgical or
pharmacological.**

**Lifelong chewing, tooth removal
or tooth movement, can change the bite
and then unbalance the jaws and jaw joints.**

**Likewise, any kind of dental work
or tooth movement can change the bite
and then rebalance the jaws and jaw joints.**

The Functional Orthodontist—1988 [266]

FJO treatment has broad potential future health applications, which are not routinely being utilized now. Many patients with middle and inner ear disorders suffer from dental problems.[267] About one-third of children have supposed ear infections, which can be reduced or eliminated by FJO dental treatment.[268] [269] A few months of FJO maxillary expansion treatment has been found to help some children suffering with chronic bed-wetting.[270] Oral devices can be effective to open airways for many patients with sleep apnea and reduce the need for throat surgeries.[271] Research shows that up to one-third of epileptics have recognizable sleep apnea, so oral devices may soon be used to treat both sleep apnea and epilepsy. [272] [273]

FJO treatment is uniquely positioned to improve overall health from birth to death.[274] FJO treatment has the unique potential to greatly influence health at any age. Few other forms of conservative, non-surgical dental or medical treatment have such broad potential. Palatal expansion, just one form of FJO therapy, shows how potent FJO techniques can be. Palatal expansion is a comparatively simple, conservative method of treatment that can be used to treat impaired nasal respiration, especially in those from age 4 through 30. Research shows it helps approximately 80 percent of mouth breathers to breath through their nose. Unique health benefits include considerable improvement in colds, respiratory infection, nasal allergy and many cases of asthma. The medical indications for palatal expansion include poor nasal airway, septal deformity, recurrent ear or nasal infection, allergic rhinitis and asthma. [275]

Consider finding an FJO dentist to improve your smile, for better general health, or just in case you need one in an emergency. FJO oral devices and treatments can uniquely improve appearance and overall body health. Non-surgical, preventive and therapeutic FJO medical dentistry proves itself, and patients say it makes good sense.

10 Reasons to Choose Functional Jaw Orthopedics
"The Newest Form of Orthodontics"

More Attractive Faces

More Beautiful Broad Smiles

**Correct Small Problems
Before They Grow Bigger**

**Fewer "Serial" Extractions
and Overall Extractions**

Active Treatment At Age 2 to 8

Adult Treatment At All Ages

Healthier Jaws & Jaw Joints—TMJs

More Balanced Bites & Jaws

Prevent Surgery

**Dental Treatment
With Positive Life Long Effects**

10 New Steps That
May Lead to Better Health:
"Save Your Teeth ~ Change Your Life"

Take 2 Multiple Vitamins With Minerals Daily (One-AM & One-PM)

Make Preventive Dental Visits Every 2-6 Months

Clean Your Mouth Well Every Day

Save Your Teeth Whenever Possible

Replace Missing Back Teeth

Wear Removable Dentures At Night

Practice Deep Nasal Breathing

Sleep with a Nasal Strip

Get a Blood Oxygen and Airway Check-up

* Find an FJO Dentist

10 New Steps That May Lead To Better Health:

1. Take Two Multiple Vitamins With Minerals Daily (One in the Morning & One at Night): Research shows vitamins are essential to health. Most of us do not eat balanced meals every day. Our bodies still require vitamins and minerals to function properly and to continuously make new cells. Some drugs cause you to lose vitamins. History teaches that a lack of just one vitamin, Vitamin C, can result in bleeding gums, tooth loss, scurvy and death. Studies show a protective effect of taking one multiple vitamin with minerals each morning and each night.

2. Make Preventive Dental Visits Every 2-6 Months: Research shows people who routinely have professional cleanings and examinations, keep more of their teeth and keep them longer. There are up to 160 tooth sides and surfaces in a mouth, and many are hard to clean. Routine dental visits every 2-6 months are just as important as homecare and fluoride efforts to keep teeth for a lifetime.

3. Clean Your Mouth Well Every Day: Research shows people who clean their mouth regularly keep their teeth the longest. Careful brushing, flossing, rinsing or water spraying all tooth surfaces takes time. It must be done well after meals, especially before sleeping.

4. Save Your Teeth Whenever Possible: Research shows those with more teeth and better tooth function are healthier. Chewing food and keeping the jaws and airway supported requires teeth. Keeping teeth requires an investment in time and money. Saving just one tooth using modern materials and techniques can take a number of dental visits and require a worthwhile investment in order to enhance personal health.

5. Replace Missing Back Teeth: Research shows that natural teeth support the jaws and airway, and promote health, so replacement of missing back teeth is important.

6. Wear Removable Dentures At Night: Research shows when teeth are missing, the jaws and airway can collapse. Denture jaw support, especially at night, is vital to keeping tongue space. Institutionalized people with fewer natural or replacement teeth (disabled, elderly, veterans, and prisoners) get sicker and die sooner than those living out of institutions.

7. Practice Deep Nasal Breathing: Research shows nasal breathing promotes good health, while mouth-breathing habits damage health. So it makes sense to practice deep nasal breathing daily. Studies now show that inhaling air through the nose helps the lungs, the heart and the whole body. Specifically, it can help asthmatics, so they need less medicine. It can reduce and reverse arteriosclerosis.

8. Sleep with a Nasal Strip: Research shows that nasal strips help improve nasal breathing for most people at night. It makes sense that regular use will be shown to improve overall health. Nasal strips flare the nostrils allowing air to be inhaled easier through fleshy passages that tend to get narrower with age.

9. Get a Blood Oxygen and Airway Check-up: Research shows that blood oxygen levels drop considerably throughout the night in some people. It makes sense to know if this is happening to you. Regular short drops in blood oxygen can affect your blood pressure and even harm you. Overnight pulse-oximetry services may be hard to find.

10. Find an FJO Doctor of Dentistry (Dentist): Research shows Functional Jaw Orthopedics differs greatly from usual dental and medical philosophies. It makes sense to find an FJO dentist in case you need one. Studies show that good dental function is significantly associated with better cognitive thought, better vision, better hearing, better lung volume, better heart volume, better muscle strength, better bone mineral content, fewer heart attacks and longer life.

Real People Stories:

The stories that follow are about real people and their real jaw and jaw-related health problems. While the individual stories are unique, the health problems and final solutions are not. Each story offers hope for those in need of alternative health care. These stories show the need for new research into areas of ignored medical dentistry.

Millions of people worldwide suffer from the health problems mentioned in the following stories. In the U.S. alone, tens of millions suffer from just chronic ear problems and headaches. Few know that conservative non-surgical jaw treatment often can help reduce or even cure their ills.

If you have health problems like those mentioned in the following real stories, you may want to seek out a provider of Functional Jaw Orthopedics. You may have to interview several dental doctors before finding one skilled in treating both the teeth and jaws. Doing so may save you time, money and pain. [see Appendix A: Where to Find FJO Providers].

If you decide to seek jaw treatment like Functional Jaw Orthopedics, remember that treatments vary, bite plate designs vary, dental provider theories of therapy vary and so do results. **Be realistic and understand while many people can be helped with FJO types of treatment, some cannot.**

**"It matters not how strait the gate,
How charged with punishments the scroll,
I am the master of my fate:
I am the captain of my soul."**

William Ernest Henley (1849-1903) [276]

Dentist Stops Ear "Infections"
Chronic Ear "Infections": Patient M. P. Age 3

My middle son was about 6 months old when he had his first ear "infection." He went on to have over 20 ear problems in just 2 ½ years. Ear problems often occurred when he was teething. Teething puts undue forces on the jaws, jaw joints, ears, and Eustachian tubes. Most of his ear problems were on one side, his right side.

Our pediatrician considered teeth and teething irrelevant. He warned that ear tubes would be recommended after the next ear event. He did not care to hear about what I saw.

I could see what the pediatrician was not trained to see. My middle son had a very narrow upper jaw—palate. His teeth erupted into his mouth in what is called a dental cross-bite. The cross-bite was on his right side, so his jaw shifted toward his right side, his right jaw joint, and his right ear.

When his next ear problem occurred, I decided to change his bite, at 3 years of age. I used dental plastic bonding materials to change and balance his bite and stop his jaw from shifting toward his right ear. He has not had another ear "infection" or problem in the 15 years since I bonded his teeth. I have learned a lot since 1987 about ears.

My middle son had chronic ear problems that my other sons did not have. His teeth caused his jaw to shift. **His "Baby TMJ" case was solved in 1987. Other FJO dentists worldwide have helped other children in the same way.**

David C. Page, D.D.S.—1987 to 2002

* The *Primary Molar Vertical Build-up* educational brochure shows this technique. (see pages 144 and 160)

My Head Pain Stopped After Dental Work

Chronic Ear & Head Problems: Patient L.A. Age 12

My mother said I had ear tubes put in my ears when I was 18 months old because of my chronic ear problems. But it took 10 more years and dental treatment to solve my constant ear problems and pain.

Even after ear tubes were placed, I still had continuous problems with my ears. They were the reason I went to the pediatrician a lot. I had drops and other stuff put in my ears, but the fluid continued to be a problem. Antibiotics didn't help. I was on antibiotics constantly. I'd take them for 10 days then stop for two days, over and over. My ENT doctor, also an allergist, couldn't help me either. He suggested allergy shots and some other things, but my mother declined.

I also had problems with headaches and felt pressure in my head, sort of like when I was in an airplane. My family traveled a lot so head pressure in an airplane was a big pain problem for me. My ears would get clogged and hurt so badly that my mother used to get hot towels from the stewardess and hold them over my ears to help. I could never get used to the pain of flying. After a flight, it took over one hour for my ears to pop and unclog and for the pain to decrease.

My ear pain and problems stopped after my dental treatment started. When I got straight teeth, I got pain free. I no longer needed to go to my doctors or take antibiotics for my ears. I remember telling my FJO dentist, **"I do not know what you did, but it's the first time I can remember not having a daily earache or headache."**

L.A.—1987

My Son Got Ear "Infections" After Dental Work

Ear and Sinus Infections: Patient M.A. Age 7

In the spring of 1998, I asked my FJO dentist why my son got ear infections after dental treatment. My son had problems all his life with his ears. I noticed he would develop a sinus and ear infection after dental visits. We also observed and photographed how just one ear would turn red on the same side of his head being treated at dental visits.

About that time my FJO dentist placed a mouth appliance to widen my son's upper jaw and bring his lower jaw forward. I began to monitor and record daily the changes in his appearance, congestion and ear fluid. I used a special ear monitor to check his ears. The findings were remarkable.

Each time a new appliance was added or adjusted, the ear monitor would change from a reading of 1-2 to 4-5 within 24 hours. The 1-2 indicated a rather normal ear and the 4-5 indicated abnormal inflammation. Ear levels would usually return to 1-3 within 2-3 days. In the beginning, these findings were often confirmed by an ENT or pediatrician being seen because of acute pain or eardrum ruptures.

By February of 1999, my son's chronic ear problems were reduced to mainly the left ear. Since September 2000, my son has been free of ear and sinus infections.

After having my son's tonsils and adenoids removed, and 5 sets of ear tubes placed, we saw only temporary improvements. We are convinced the orthodontic approach has had the most positive effect on reducing his once-chronic ear and sinus infections.

M.A.'s Mother—2001

A Soft Bite Plate Stopped My Morning Pain

Morning Headaches, Earaches: Patient J.I. Age 34

One morning, over a year ago, I woke up with severe pain in my right jaw. The pain went up to my right ear. I couldn't open my jaw wide enough to even take an aspirin. I had to go on a liquid diet for a while. It took about 3½ weeks for my jaw to feel better. My morning headaches, earaches and face pain continued to bother me.

Eventually I went to a dentist. He told me I needed a lot of crown work and fillings replaced. He first sent me to an orthodontist who told me to have my wisdom teeth removed and then he would move my teeth and restructure my bite. It was a lot of work to do, so I waited awhile.

For about a year, I woke up daily with a headache, mostly on my right side. I had right ear pain in the morning, my right jaw and jaw joints hurt, and my jaw clicked and popped. My right ear and sinuses were constantly congested.

I decided to get another opinion from my hometown FJO dentist. He made me a soft bite plate appliance, which made a big difference in 3-4 days. I've been wearing the soft bite plate now for 3 months. I know it helps. I wear it every night. Sometimes I even wear it during the day, especially if I feel tense or know I am grinding my teeth.

My jaw pain and headaches are gone. I wear my bite plate every night because it works and because I have gotten so much relief from it. It only took about a day to get used to it. I did not need new crowns placed, fillings replaced, orthodontic treatment or teeth removed.

J.I.—1998

Death Knocks When the Lower Jaw Drops
Low Overnight Oxygen: M.P. Age 18 and W.M. Age 66

M.P. was diagnosed with obstructive sleep apnea (OSA) at the very early age of 18, after going through an overnight sleep study. M.P. had the recommended uvula removal surgery (UPPP) but within a few months, his wife said he again slept like he still had OSA. M.P. also noticed he was tired again during the day. So we made him a custom dental device to hold his lower jaw forward during sleep. Then we checked his oxygen levels with an overnight oxygen meter called a **Memory Pulse-Oximeter**. What we found was quite amazing. After the throat surgery, without a mouthpiece, M.P. had 143 blood oxygen dips of at least 3% for at least six seconds through a night's sleep. Wearing a dental mouthpiece cut the dips in half to 74. **Wearing a mouthpiece and a nasal strip cut the oxygen dips from 143 to 32, a more acceptable level to support his health by raising his blood oxygen levels.**

W.M. had just a top denture and his left leg would swell at night at the age of 66. His daughter-in-law, a dental assistant, thought his night oxygen levels should be checked, so we did a little investigation. **We found W.M. was lucky to live through a night's sleep.** With his top full denture in place, W.M.'s blood oxygen level would drop to about 60% off and on through the night. In a hospital, if he went below 94%, he would probably be put on tank oxygen. It was the overnight results without his denture that supported a major study indicating people with dentures should go against a century of advice and now wear their dentures at night. **Without his denture, his blood oxygen dipped to an unbelievable 20%. He was lucky to live through the night! His physician was advised of the results, and a sleep study was then scheduled.**

One Little Bite Plate Took Away 30 Years of Pain

Chronic Headaches, Insomnia: Patient J.W. Age 46

The difference in my life has been dramatic since using the new bite plates my FJO dentist made for me. I've never really documented all the things that have bothered me for years because it makes me feel like a whiner and complainer.

Quite honestly, when I did discuss some of these things with various physicians, you could literally see their eyes glaze over.

I had a severe overbite as a child. Five years, three states and three orthodontists later, I still do not think my bite is right. I now have a very small mouth and a deep bite, so my lower teeth constantly rub the roof of my mouth raw.

My headaches and insomnia started in junior high. The ophthalmic migraines were like a non-stop light show.

I went to the college infirmary and received medication in the early '70s and have been taking some kind or another ever since.

About 20 years ago, in the early '80s, I met my husband and started coming to your practice.

Eleven and one-half years ago I gave birth to triplets. Many of the symptoms I experience were attributed to this.

I was seeing one of your associates and was in a high-stress position at work. Your associate constructed a bite plate for me to relieve my jaw pain. It helped the roof of my mouth and some of the jaw pain caused by grinding.

But I still had vertigo, constant ear congestion and aches, and sinus infections which became a way of life. Then came early menopause and middle age. I thought I was aging fast.

I wore my old bite plate until almost two years ago, when you took over the care of my teeth.

When you made the soft plate, I was thrilled in the decrease in ear congestion and the ability to sleep most of the night. Because it was a soft plate, the grinding was absorbed by it and the jaw pain disappeared. My migraines dropped to one or two a month.

When you first made a hard bite plate to use long term, I didn't like it. After using it for a while, I noticed I could sleep all night. Now I am able to stay awake all day.

The cycle has been broken and I'm not constantly tired. Consequently, I now have the energy to exercise, thereby losing some weight.

The vertigo has been almost completely eliminated, and I've had one sinus infection in 18 months, as opposed to six or seven a year.

As long as I use the bite plate, I do not have the earaches and a waxy sensation. I had only one migraine in the last four months. That's a miracle in my book.

I know I may need further treatment to stabilize my bite, but the bite plates are keeping me comfortable right now.

Thank you so much for your humor and understanding and for solving so many problems with one little bite dental plate appliance!

J.W.—2001

Nothing Helped My Head Like the Bite Plate

Migraines, Dizziness, Vertigo: Patient M.C. Age 47

I was in pain for over five years. Flying in airplanes made me feel worse for a month after a flight. I started out with headaches at first and then the ear pain came. My ears felt stuffy most of the time. My right ear was the worst; it felt completely stuffed up; it got much worse on airplane flights.

I had some dizziness, loss of equilibrium and fainting spells. I'd be standing up, and then all of a sudden, I would tilt one way or the other. I'd have to find something to hold onto. It only lasted a few seconds, but it was still there.

About a month ago, I saw my FJO dentist for dental jaw treatment. He examined me, did some tests and took some x-rays. He said he thought he could help me, so he made me a plastic bite plate to wear all the time. The bite plate kept my teeth apart.

After wearing the bite plate for only about an hour, I noticed some difference. The right ear started to become a little clearer. After I had it in for three days, I had no more ear pain, no stuffiness, and no dizziness. I remember saying, "You're not going to believe this, but I can feel the ear pressure diminishing." I remember rating most of my problems a 10 (very bad) on a scale of 1 to 10. Now just one month later they are all zero; they are gone.

The last time I was on an airplane flight, I had severe ear pain in the right ear. After a very long flight, it took me a month just to get over the pressure of the ear. The flight was about eight hours long. Since then, I started taking shorter flights, like an hour or two. I would still always have pain.

I was scheduled to go on this trans-Atlantic flight three weeks ago. I was terrified because I knew I was going to have this pain and just didn't know what to do about it. So I tried the bite plate and it worked.

I just came back a few hours ago after another eight-hour flight and had no pain at all. Flying out and then back, I had no pain, no pressure, no stuffiness, no ear pressure, no nothing. I felt fantastic. I must have told 50 people how I feel 100% better. I feel better than I have felt in five years.

The bite plate definitely helped me after nothing else did. I had been to five or six different physicians over the course of five years: family doctors; internist; eye doctor; ear, nose and throat physician; and a neurologist. All of them prescribed medication or treatment such as exercise or getting glasses.

It took about a week to get used to the plastic bite plate. At first, I thought I would never get used to it, even though I knew it was helping and even though it would relieve the pressure. It was a little bit uncomfortable. Then after a day or two, I didn't even notice it. I feel so much better with it in.

If I forget to wear the appliance, I definitely have pressure. I've only slept without it one night, when I was on vacation and forgot to put it in after a very late night. I woke up during the night, grinding my teeth and there was pain in my ear. I thought, "Oh no, I am doing this with the appliance in too?" Then I realized I didn't have it in. I was grinding my teeth and my ear was definitely in pain. So I got up and put it in, and that was the end of it.

The dental bite plate definitely made me feel better. It keeps my teeth apart and my lower jaw forward.

M.C.—1987

Surgery Through My Brain Was One Option

Meniere's Disease, 2 ½ Years: Patient C.E. Age 47

T wo years ago, I started having problems with ringing in my ear, then daily vertigo attacks. I went to a series of doctors and specialists in different states. Each had a different diagnosis for my problem.

I went to an Ear Nose and Throat specialist who diagnosed my symptoms as being Meniere's disease. He gave me strong medication and monitored me for about a year and a half. My symptoms continued to get worse. The daily vertigo attacks became pretty severe.

Next, I went to a specialist in Pennsylvania. After a series of tests, I was offered three surgical treatment options to choose from. They said although treatment might not make my symptoms go away, it might make the daily vertigo attacks less severe, and hopefully help me. I thought about the options for six months. The options they gave me to choose from involved major risks.

The first treatment option included some injections into my eardrum that would hopefully deaden the balance nerve. The success rate of that treatment wasn't really great, so they were not really sure if it would work.

The second option involved surgically going in behind my ear and severing some of the balance nerves. Risks included the possibility of severing nerves that controlled the facial muscles. I might then need some rehabilitation, even learning to walk again, stuff like that.

The third option involved going in and lifting my brain up and severing the nerves that way. The risk in that was stroke. It also could require about six months of rehabilitation to learn to walk again. Each suggested treatment involved quite a bit of risk. The procedures evidently were not fool-proof.

During that six-month period, I thought about what I needed to do and what I should do. That spring, the vertigo attacks became more severe. Sometimes I'd have two a day. It really made it difficult to go to work and do my job. I didn't know when an attack would happen.

I needed some dental work, so I came to an FJO dentist. At one of my dental visits, I told him I had to delay further dental work awhile. I had to have one of the procedures done for the Meniere's disease, which was getting worse.

I told the dentist what I had gone through the last couple of years. He said he thought he could help me. He explained how the jaws can control a lot of things. We discussed how an ill-fitting dental crown placed before my problems began probably shifted my bite and jaws. So he made two bite plates to balance my bite and jaws — one to wear during the day and another design for use at night.

* Immediately after starting this treatment, the symptoms went away. I haven't had a vertigo attack since I started wearing the bite guards three years ago. The ringing in my ears, a part of the Meniere's disease, has greatly been reduced. I no longer have earaches in my left ear. Hearing tests showed that I had a 75% loss in my left ear. Now I have days where the hearing is just as good as it is in my right ear. **Dental bite plates certainly made a difference in my life, and a second phase of treatment keeps my jaw balanced.**

C.E.—2001

* The *Meniere's Disease and Dental Care* educational video shows this patient. (see pages 145 and 160)

My Wife Likes My Dental Device: It Changed My Life

Snoring, Sleep Apnea, Tired: Patient C.F. Age 54

Waking up in the morning felt like coming back from the dead. It didn't matter whether I would sleep for five or eight hours. I would feel dizzy very often upon arising. I'd shake it off after a hot shower.

Sleep for me was never sound, and breathing was always through my mouth due to sinus problems.

During the day, there were episodes when I lacked concentration and felt more tired than I should.

My wife pointed out frequently that during the night, I would snore, stop breathing and my chest would heave, as though I was trying to breath but couldn't. This was followed by violent jerks, which would cause me to shift positions and begin breathing again. She believed that I had sleep apnea and should consult a physician.

During a spring physical, I finally related my wife's story and was referred to a pulmonologist and subsequently a sleep study. The results of this study confirmed that I had sleep apnea. I was averaging 25 episodes per hour lasting from 12 to 30 seconds, where I was not breathing. My oxygen level was falling to 87% (below a desired 94% minimum of blood oxygen).

The pulmonologist suggested possible solutions including surgery and a machine with a tethered sleeping-mask called a CPAP that would force air into my lungs.

When I told the doctor that I first wanted to try something my dentist had suggested, he looked surprised.

I work in the medical field so I did some research on sleep apnea treatments on my own.

I felt that surgery was out of the question, based on my research and the poor results reported for surgical intervention in sleep apnea.

Furthermore, I knew it was not realistic for me to sleep each night with a hose strapped to my face that was connected to a machine. So I told the doctor that I would first try the dental device and if it did not work, I would be back.

Our family dentist, also an FJO dentist, fabricated a custom oral snore appliance in only one office visit. I began using the mouthpiece and was amazed at the results.

Very quickly I was sleeping better and had more energy the next day. I also found I was now breathing through my nose more, because I would wake up with my mouth closed.

Every now and then I get lazy and forget my oral appliance. Well, if I am not awakened at night by my wife, she certainly lets me know the next morning – "You didn't sleep with your mouthpiece in did you? I was awake half the night with your snoring and gasping."

I just came off of one of my lazy periods and returned to using the oral appliance again this week. I slept through the night last night and didn't even get up in the middle of the night to visit the bathroom!

FJO dentistry helped change my life with an oral appliance. I am sleeping better and so is my wife. Simply put, the bite plate works.

C.F.—2001

I Had Eye Pain From My Jaws
Acute Left Eye & Head Pain: Patient J.N. Age 64

Several months ago, I began having very intense pain in my left eye. It always started at night. The pain was always concentrated at my left eye, where it began. Pain would spread to the left ear and my left side. I had headaches, eye pain, ear pain, face pain, neck pain, back pain, tight neck, ear congestion, sinus congestion, and a few teeth that hurt, all on my left side.

The pain was so intense the only thing I could do to get relief was go to bed and try to sleep. But I couldn't sleep. The pain would last 7-8 hours and sometimes I'd get nauseated. I thought it was a bad case of a sinus infection, cluster headaches or maybe a migraine.

My family doctor thought I might have cluster headaches. He prescribed sinus medication and a painkiller. Neither drug did any good. The intense pain continued every night for about two weeks.

I went to my general dentist to check for tooth abscesses, but none were found. He did find evidence of TMJ disorder. We discussed how it might be causing my pain.

I went to my eye doctor to see if there was anything wrong with my eye; there was not. He referred me to an ear specialist who checked and found nothing wrong with my ear. The ear doctor did agree there were symptoms of TMJ.

An FJO dentist made some bite plates for me. The first one took my pain from a 9 (on a scale of 1-10) down to 3-4. **A second bite plate made the pain disappear after three adjustments balanced my bite. Now I am pain free again.**

J.N.—1987

I Was Dizzy, Now I Am a Believer
Mysterious Dizzy Spells; Patient B.S. Age 74

In August of 1999, I began to experience dizzy spells. When I laid down in bed and turned on my left side the room would spin violently. It's called vertigo. The spinning would stop when I laid on my back or on my right side. The room would start to spin again when I would look up over my head to work or just to look.

I went to my physician internist who sent me to an ear, nose & throat specialist (ENT). They made several tests of my eyes and ears and found nothing. I was given a medicine, which had little if any effect. I was told there was nothing to do but hope that the problem would pass. They really did not know what was causing the problem.

Twenty-five years earlier, I had a similar problem, which they called Meniere's disease. It lasted about two months and went away. This time the problems did not go away. In fact they were lingering and affecting my life.

In March of 2000, I saw an FJO dentist who took a mold of my lower teeth. He made a mouthpiece, which changed my bite. I wore the mouthpiece 48 hours straight and soon discovered I could turn any way I wanted in bed without any dizziness. This change occurred rather quickly. I have been wearing the mouthpiece ever since then, except when I eat. I have not had even one dizzy spell.

I am amazed at how well this worked. I am a believer. I am also eternally grateful someone was willing to help a 74-year-old man regain his confidence in living.

B.S.—2001

Dentist Stops Daughter's Ear "Infections"

Letter From Dr. Steven Fink: Daughter S.F. Age 5½

Dear Dr. Page: I visited you in October of 1999 to discuss my daughter and her ear problems. Her medical history was routine except for the presence of retained fluid in both of her ears. She was diagnosed with ear infections that were treated with various antibiotics on: 9/94, 12/94, 1/95, 2/95, 12/97, 10/98, 3/99 and 7/99.

After the last ear infection in 7/99, her pediatrician referred her to an ear, nose and throat specialist (ENT). He examined her and said she needed surgically placed ear drain tubes immediately. We went to a Doctor of Osteopathy (DO) friend for a second opinion. A hearing test determined she was suffering from a decrease in hearing. He then referred her to a second ENT specialist who said ear tube surgery was appropriate but could be delayed if we put her on a course of drugs and observed her frequently.

My daughter had a deep bite with her lower permanent incisors erupting behind her lower baby teeth. Since her baby teeth would not loosen, the conventional treatment was to extract them. I was uncomfortable with that option (serial extractions). I could see there was already not enough space for the other new teeth to fit in.

I remembered reading one of your articles in the *Functional Orthodontist Journal* about ear infections among other dental/medical problems. I also discovered a one-day course you were teaching on the subjects. After contacting you, you were kind enough to set up a consultation with me and my daughter's study models, photos and x-rays. You immediately recognized her lower jaw (mandible) was trapped behind her upper jaw (maxilla).

To make room for her lower incisors and relieve her ears, you recommended a simple course of combined treatment. You advised an upper removable palatal expansion appliance to be worn actively for about three months, and then passively for about three months and dental composite bonding (plastic material) on the lower baby molars.

*At the same time, you advised that a lower composite bonded "ramp" buildup be placed to immediately open the deep dental bite. You explained it as "braces-without-braces" bonding to change the jaw position as new teeth erupted. All of this was done, with my own modification of the composite bite ramps. I used an indirect method. This allowed easy placement on my young daughter.

My daughter is now about 7 years old. Truth be told, her permanent molars are all in now and the indirect composites are still undisturbed after more than a year!

I admit I was skeptical when you told me this would make room for her teeth and may stop the ear infections. Her last antibiotic for an ear infection was 7/99. Her treatment began in 11/99 and ran for six months leaving the composite buildups in place. You were right! (Of course you knew that!) Thank you for your outstanding clinical diagnosis, and I hope these results help spread your message.

The most exciting part of all of this is that we never elected to have surgical ear drain tubes placed, and my daughter lost her two lower primary centrals without dental extractions. In addition, her chronic ear infections stopped after having the treatment you recommended.

Stephen Fink, DMD—2001

* The *Primary Molar Vertical Build-up* educational brochure shows this technique. (see pages 144 and 160)

Importance of Breastfeeding
Letter From Dr. Brian Palmer—Kansas City, MO

After over 25 years of research, and one year of developing my website, I recently posted my final presentation—**The Importance of Breastfeeding as it Relates to Total Health.** It is a 268-slide presentation in Acrobat Reader format, in three parts for easier opening.

The format should allow anyone in the world to view it. I am hoping the material will help educate many other health care providers, especially pediatricians. In the presentation, I try to demonstrate how breastfeeding reduces the risk of many health problems in our society. Millions of dollars in health care costs could be saved just by breastfeeding and understanding the severe consequences of some infant habits.

The presentation addresses frequently asked questions, such as: What are rugae and what is their purpose during the act of breastfeeding? What is Obligate Nose Breathing and how does it impact breastfeeding? Why is breastfeeding so important for the proper development of the oral cavity and airway? What are the consequences of a tongue thrust? What are bubble palates and how can they impact breastfeeding? Why does tongue-tie cause sore breasts? What damage can excessive infant habits cause? Why are breastfed babies prettier? **How does breastfeeding reduce the risk of obstructive sleep apnea, long face syndrome, Sudden Infant Death Syndrome (SIDS), otitis media, obesity and cancer?**

When viewers have seen the final presentation, I encourage them to go back over the other presentations and articles on the website, especially the presentation on sleep apnea. They should then have more meaning.

Breastfeeding should be elevated to a new level of importance once the medical community and general public understand the importance of breastfeeding, as it relates to reducing sleep apnea and adult illness.

* The health of an infant begins with a healthy pregnant mother. After birth, the health of the child continues with breastfeeding, which greatly influences the development of the human jaws and airway.

Seven years ago, my brother, five years my senior, had a massive stroke. It is believed his stroke was secondary to sleep apnea. He is now confined to a long-term care facility with little hope of ever leaving. He is but one example of how early diagnosis and treatment could possibly have prevented this tragedy. Cost to the health care system for this one case has been significant.

Over 40 years ago I promised myself I would try to do something to make the world a better place. I feel my website fulfills that promise. The burden of that promise has now been lifted from my shoulders. I feel I have done the best that I can.

I only hope others who have the funding will continue my research. Please share this note with others: For Better Health. It is now time for me to play more golf and walk the beaches with my lovely wife.

Dr. Brian Palmer—2002

Web: www.brianpalmerdds.com

* The *Functional Jaw Orthopedics* educational brochure shows the negative effects of not breastfeeding. (see pages 145 and 160)

"There are three parts in truth:
first, the inquiry, which is the wooing of it;
secondly, the knowledge of it, which is the
presence of it; and thirdly, the belief,
which is the enjoyment of it."

Francis Bacon (1561-1626) [277]

Medical Dentistry Now

Letter From Dr. Derek Mahony—Sydney, Australia

Recurrent Otitis Media: Mother K.B. of Patient Age 7

Fortunately, a family friend advised us to see Dr. Mahony. "My child had recurrent middle ear infections for many years and my local physician kept prescribing antibiotics. Out of frustration, we sought the opinion of an ENT specialist. He advocated placing ear tubes. Dr. Mahony recommended a non-surgical, non-medicated approach of upper arch (jaw) expansion. This was extremely effective. Joanna, our daughter, has not had middle ear problems for the last four years. Her ENT specialist is also amazed at the improvement of her hearing after upper jaw expansion."

Moderate Obstructive Sleep Apnea: Patient S.M. Age 45

I was diagnosed by my respiratory physician as having mild obstructive sleep apnea. My wife couldn't sleep next to me due to my loud snoring. I was always tired at work and never slept well throughout the night. My physician recommended use of a CPAP machine or surgical intervention. Neither of these options appealed to me so I sought the opinion of Dr. Mahony. He had treated our neighbor for a similar condition. After reviewing my sleep study data, he prescribed an orthotic appliance (a dental device) that postured my lower jaw forward when I was asleep. This treatment was extremely successful and avoided the need for surgery as well as the discomfort associated with the CPAP machine. I have stopped snoring and now my wife and I both have a better night's rest. My respiratory physician was amazed at the reduction of my RDI after the use of this "snoring appliance" and now recommends that his patients try a jaw re-positioning appliance before embarking on more invasive treatment modalities.

**In the year 2000,
healthcare costs in the U.S.
soared to $1.3 trillion.**

Department of Health and Human Services [278]

**In the year 2000,
only about 5% of all U.S.
health-care expenditures, $60 billion,
were for private practice dental services.**

**About half of the cost was paid "out-of-pocket"
and about half from private dental insurance.**

Less than 5% came from government sources.

American Dental Association News—2002 [279]

**Alternative medicine is becoming more popular
among consumers and prescribed more
by health care professionals.**

The Health Care Manager—2002 [280]

EPILOGUE: 12 Steps to Future Medical Dentistry

B y now you have either dropped your jaw or dropped this book which gives only a glimpse of what may lie ahead. Future medical dentistry and healthcare is literally in your hands. It contains powerful information for you to use. If you want access to alternative medical dentistry and unique alternative care providers, you must take active action. **To help influence the future direction of healthcare consider taking these 12 steps:**

1. Research your own healthcare needs and passionately search out your treatment options and choices. Once you learn where to find healthcare information you will be amazed at what you discover. [see page 140-141]

2. Organize efforts to expand alternative healthcare options, especially at institutions receiving public funding. Alternative healthcare is often called complimentary care, and then treated as a second healing option. Alternative care can be the best primary treatment and not the second option. Furthermore, it is often better than drugs or surgery.

3. Organize efforts to teach all healthcare providers an overview of medical dentistry and the unique health benefits.

4. Organize efforts to set up model medical dentistry centers. Unique medical dentistry can only be delivered efficiently in a unique environment. People can only receive medical dentistry in a special setting. These centers must be designed to deliver total dental care. They must also have examination rooms for the needed healthcare providers: FJO dentist, pediatrician, internist, sleep medicine specialist, otolaryngologist and others.

**Acute dental conditions result in about
2.5 million work days lost,
4.6 million bed days, and
9.7. million days of restricted activity.**

US Dept of Health and Human Services—2000 [281]

**The evidence is overwhelming that oral infections
have a profound effect on oral health,
general health, quality of life,
and economic well-being.**

Compendium—2002 [282]

**Medical research papers commonly contain
methodological errors, report results selectively,
and draw unjustified conclusions.**

**The aim of medical research should be to
advance scientific knowledge and either directly
or indirectly lead to improvements in the
treatment and prevention of disease.**

Journal of the American Medical Association—2002 [283]

5. Organize efforts to change health benefits and payment approaches. People need health benefits to be a benefit and cover valuable alternative treatments like medical dentistry. Dental insurance benefits have not changed much since 1980: plan maximums are still $500-1500; deductibles are from $10-50 (often per person); and the list of plan exclusions can now exceed the number of procedures many dentists perform. Dental insurance has been used somewhat as bait (a loss-leader) to steer people into medical plans and to providers on lists. This must change because $1 spent on medical dentistry may save up to $100 in medical costs. Insurance restrictions and the value of alternative care force consumers to spend billions of dollars out-of-pocket yearly.

6. Organize efforts to redirect publicly funded research. Billions of public tax dollars should go to areas that in time benefit the public more than those doing the research.[284]

7. Organize efforts to review and revamp published and unpublished medical research. Nearly 50% of published medical journal articles allegedly contain bias. Additionally, research studies with positive outcomes have a much higher chance of being published than those with negative outcomes.[285] Throughout history, the scientific world has used negative results to help determine and direct future research. Because hundreds of thousands of negative study conclusions have never been published, billions of research dollars have been wasted. This is a tragic loss to progress and to society.

8. Support and advocate exclusive breast-feeding for about 6-12 months. It is best for most children (excluding those with mothers on drugs, etc.) You can impact the health of the next generation and reduce overall health care costs.

9. Organize and lead lawsuit reform efforts. We are suing experienced healthcare providers and quality businesses out of existence. Jury awards must become reasonable if the art and science of medicine is to survive.

**Throughout recorded history
the dental ills of mankind have been treated
by medical specialists particularly
associated with surgery.**

**However, deep-rooted cultural tradition
relegated surgeons and those engaged in the
dental art to a class deemed socially,
intellectually and economically inferior to that of
the physician, causing widespread neglect of
dentistry until the 16th century.**

*American Academy of the History of Dentistry
Journal of the History of Dentistry*—1998 [286]

10. Organize efforts to teach and support dentists interested in learning and then providing FJO dentistry. Current teaching institutions cannot teach what they do not know. Dental schools, even those that espouse research, are having trouble preparing dental graduates to perform satisfactory general dentistry. They are light years behind the knowledge and skills needed for FJO dentistry. This past year, allegedly over 50% of the graduates at one dental school failed their dental board exam the first time, and some needed to take the test three times before passing. Another school announced plans to add a fifth year to their dental program and totally bypass dental licensure testing.[287]

Dentists that choose to practice FJO medical dentistry must have good reason (money and respect) because it takes extraordinary learning and lots of hard work. If patients want medical dentistry, they must finally view dental doctors and their staffs with the respect they are due. Patients and dentists together must demand change and new approaches from the whole healthcare system. They must also understand that needed changes will take considerable time.

11. Support efforts by dentists to change state laws that restrict the scope of dental practice and prevent dentists from advertising alternative medical dentistry services. The scope of dental practice currently does not allow dentists to advertise, prescribe or deliver dental care as treatment for medical reasons. The American Dental Association Code of Ethics calls upon dentists to follow high ethical standards, which have the benefit of the patient as their primary goal: "Do No Harm and Do Good." It also warns dentists not to violate the dental code.[288] If patients want new medical dentistry, they must demand it along with the political and legal changes necessary to make it available.

12. Consider sending this book *Your Jaws ~ Your Life,* to family, friends, politicians, and dental/medical authorities. This key step will advance medical dentistry the fastest.

**"Knowledge is of two kinds.
We know a subject ourselves,
or we know where we can
find information upon it."**

Samuel Johnson (1709-1784) [289]

APPENDIX A:

Where to Find FJO Dentists

DISCLAIMER: The following organizations have stated an interest in the jaws, so their members should have some knowledge of functional jaw orthopedics. There is no implied or explicit endorsement of any group, any individual practitioner or his/her services, by the author or publisher of **Your Jaws ~ Your Life.** There are other organizations and dentists who have an understanding of functional jaw orthopedics and sleep apnea treatments and philosophies. It is important to understand that a true FJO dentist believes that changing teeth can change how the upper and lower jaws relate and interact. Some tooth changes that can cause jaw changes include bite plates, braces, dentures, crowns, bridgework, fillings, extractions and bite adjustments.

American Association for Functional Orthodontics
Publishers of: *The Functional Orthodontist*
A Journal of Functional Jaw Orthopedics
AAFO, 106 South Kent Street
Winchester, Virginia 22601 USA
www.aafo.org

American Academy of Craniofacial Pain
AACP: 520 W. Pipeline Road,
Hurst Texas 76053 USA
www.aahnfp.org

Society for the Study of Cranio-Mandibular Disorders.
International and U.K.
www.JawAche.com

The Cranio Group
International and U.K.
www.CranioGroup.com

APPENDIX B:

How to Search PubMed®
A Major Health Information Resource

One of the greatest resources for finding health related information is the PubMed© medical database, which is maintained by the U.S. Government. You might consider learning how to access this vast health information resource.

The National Library of Medicine PubMed© web site stores and organizes health articles and research summaries, known as abstracts, from around the world. These abstracts often have study content or conclusions that can be understood by those without medical training. You might be amazed at how fascinating one sentence, from one abstract, taken from a lengthy multi-million dollar study can be.

The U.S. Government National Institute of Health (NIH) makes the PubMed© database of over 11 million health articles available to the public. Internet access to the PubMed© database is available at: **www.PubMed.gov.**

The PubMed© database has special terms for use and you should read them in the disclaimer and copyright section.

The National Library of Medicine (NLM) site Medical Information Disclaimer is worth noting:

> "It is not the intention of NLM to provide specific medical advice, but rather to provide users with information to better understand their health and their diagnosed disorders. Specific medical advice will not be provided, and NLM urges you to consult with a qualified physician for diagnosis and for answers to your personal questions."

An Example of How to Use PubMed®:

To read about the *tonsils,* the *heart, cor pulmonale* (heart en-largement) and effects of *tonsillectomy* (tonsil removal):

1) Go to **www.PubMed.gov**
2) In the search topic box type the word *"tonsils"*
3) Select "Go"
   A list of about <u>6400</u> articles should appear.
   You can now read for days about the tonsils.

4) In the search topic box add the word *"heart"*
5) Select "Go" to refine the article list.
   The list should now focus on about <u>145</u> articles.
   You can now read about the tonsils and heart.

6) In the topic box add the word *"cor pulmonale"*
   the medical term for right heart enlargement
7) Select "Go" to further refine the article list.
   The list should now show about <u>43</u> articles.
   You can now read about tonsils & heart enlargement.

8) In the topic box add the word *"tonsillectomy"*
9) Select "Go" to further refine the article list.
   The list should now show about <u>25</u> articles.
   You can now read about a health option for those that may have heart damage from enlarged tonsils.

Note: Many articles on the database contain no abstract, so you would have to go to a health library to read the article abstract summary or the whole article itself.

Caution: Bias in medical literature has been reported to be present in as many as half (50%) of all published articles. So read for information, but routinely seek your doctor's advice.

APPENDIX C:

Suggested Reading for
The Public & Health Care Professionals:

Functional Jaw Orthopedics
www.SmilePage.com and www.AAFO.org

Airway, Breast Feeding & Sleep Apnea:
www.BrianPalmerDDS.com

Dental Treatment for Otitis Media:
www.DrBranam.com

Diet, Nutrition and Body Health:
www.Price-Pottenger.org

11 Million Health Research Summaries:
www.PubMed.gov

Book: Nutrition and Physical Degeneration
by Weston A. Price D.D.S.
A powerful book of strong evidence and photographs, from
Dr. Price's 1920s-1930s worldwide research, that shows
the adverse effects of the modern diet.

APPENDIX D:

Additional Reading for Health Care Professionals:

The Functional Orthodontist (Quarterly)
Journal of the American Association for Functional
Orthodontics by various AAFO Authors
Valuable Individual Article Reprints Available

**Maxillofacial Orthopedics: A Clinical Approach for the
Growing Child:** by Ahlin/White/Tsamtsouris/Saadia
An excellent book which explains the orthopedic view and
need for more comprehensive malocclusion correction.

Essentials of Facial Growth by Enlow and Hans
A superb book on jaw & skull growth and development.

Oral Motor Assessment and Treatment: Ages and Stages
by Diane Chapman Bahr, MS, CCC-SLP
A professional speech & language book resource.

Facial Growth and Facial Orthopedics by Van der Linden
This book shows facial growth and development, and the
benefits of facial-orthopedics, in a clear and concise manner.

A Four Book Orthodontic/Orthopedic Series: by Gill B.
Bastein, D.M.D. and J. W. "Skip" Truitt, Jr., B.S., D.D.S.
Four easy to read books teach one excellent FJO approach.
1-Applied Functional Orthopedic & Orthodontic Therapy
2-Applied Orthodontic Therapy: The Straight Arch Appliance
3-The Bimler Cephalometric Analysis
4-Advanced Orthopedic and Orthodontic Therapy

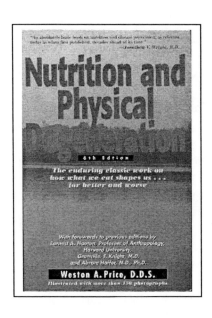

Nutrition and Physical Degeneration
Book by
Weston A Price, D.D.S.

"The enduring classic work on how what we eat shapes us...for better and worse."

Paperback: 526 pages, With great illustrations!

$19.95

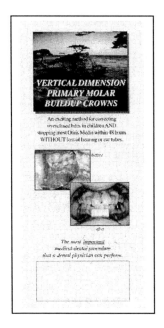

Vertical Dimension Primary Molar Buildup Crowns
Tri-fold
Patient Education Brochure

"An exciting method for correcting over-closed bites in children, and stopping most otitis media within 48 hours, without loss of hearing or ear tubes."

$5 per mini-pack of 10

See Product ***Quick Order Form*** on Page 160

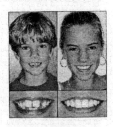

FUNCTIONAL JAW ORTHOPEDICS

NEW
Early Orthodontics
Starting at Birth

Functional Jaw Orthopedics (FJO) is the newest, most progressive form of orthodontic treatment. This approach treats teeth and jaws starting at birth to manage growth, development and deformation. With this method, various dental techniques are used in one or more phases of treatment to give patients beautiful broad healthy smiles.

**Functional
Jaw Orthopedics**
Tri-fold
Patient Education Brochure

New
Early Orthodontics
Starting at Birth
(Breastfeeding)

www.SmilePage.com

$5 per mini-pack of 10

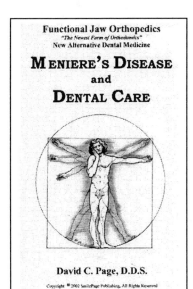

Functional Jaw Orthopedics
"The Newest Form of Orthodontics"
New Alternative Dental Medicine
**MENIERE'S DISEASE
and
DENTAL CARE**

David C. Page, D.D.S.

Copyright © 2002 SmilePage Publishing, All Rights Reserved

**Meniere's Disease
and
Dental Care**
Patient Education—Testimonial
12 Minute
VHS Video

*Learn what is not known about
Meniere's disease...
...see how dental treatment
helped one patient
avoid drugs and surgery.*

$19.95

See Product *Quick Order Form* on Page 160

End Note References

1 Bradley, J.P., Daniels, L.F., Jones, T.C. (1975). International Encyclopedia of Quotations, J. G. Ferguson Publishing Company. p. 735.

2 Ibid. p. 734.

3 Center for Disease Control, Associated Press, Baltimore Sun 3/99

4 Coronary heart disease mortality trends among whites and blacks—Appalachia and United States, 1980-1993. MMWR Morb Mortal Wkly Rep 1998 Nov 27;47(46):1005-8,1015.

5 The New Webster's Comprehensive Dictionary of the English Language. American International Press. 1985 p. BT-80.

6 Ibid. p. BT-69.

7 Dudley DL, Pitts-Poarch AR. Psychophysiologic aspects of respiratory control. Clin Chest Med 1980 Jan;1(1):131-43.

8 Bradley, J.P., Daniels, L.F., Jones, T.C. (1975) The International Encyclopedia of Quotations, J.G. Ferguson Publishing Company. p. 527.

9 Ibid.

10 The New Webster's Comprehensive Dictionary of the English Language. American International Press. 1985 p. BT-67.

11 Ibid.

12 Ibid.

13 Vitruvius on Architecture—Book VIII, 1st Century B.C.

14 CPR for Family and Friends. American Heart Association. 2000 pp.6-7.

15 Lim BL. Airway management-when and how? Singapore Med J 2001 Sep;Suppl 1:043-5.

16 Buckner F. Is there an alternative medicine clinic in your future? J Med Pract Manage 1999 Mar-Apr;14(5):263-7.

17 World Health Organization Report 2000.

18 www.quotationspage.com

19 Page, DC. The new dental-medical renaissance. Medically efficacious functional jaw orthopedics. Funct Orthod 1999 Jan-Mar;16(1):16-22, 24-5.

20 Manchanda SC, Narang R, Reddy KS, Sachdeva U, Prabhakaran D, Dharmanand S, Rajani M, Bijlani R. Retardation of coronary atherosclerosis with yoga lifestyle intervention. J Assoc Physicians India 2000 Jul;48:687-94.

21 http://www.leonardo2002.de/ehome/egeheim.html

22 Ring, Malvin E. Dentistry An Illustrated History. Harry N. Abrams, Inc. Publishers 1985. Royal Library of Assyrian King Ashurbanipal. 1700 B.C.

23 Matthew 24:51. New Living Translation Bible. Tyndale House Publishers.

24 House JS. Understanding social factors and inequalities in health: 20th century progress and 21st century prospects. J Health Soc Behav 2002 Jun;43(2):125-42.

25 Bahr DC. Oral Motor Assessment and treatment: ages and stages. Allyn & Bacon. p. 73.

26 Ring, Malvin E. Dentistry An Illustrated History. Harry N. Abrams, Inc. Publishers. 1985.

27 Luke 13:28. New Living Translation Bible. Tyndale House Publishers.

28 Van der Linden, Frans P.G.M. Facial Growth and Facial Orthopedics. Quintessence Publishing Co. 1986.

29 Page DC. Breastfeeding is early functional jaw orthopedics (an introduction). Funct Orthod 2001 Fall;18(3):24-7.

[30] Ahlin J. H., White G. E., Tsamtsouris A., Saadia M. Maxillofacial Orthopedics: A Clinical Approach for the Growing Child. 1984

[31] Ohm E, Silness J. Size of the mandibular jaw angle related to age, tooth retention and gender. J Oral Rehabil 1999 Nov;26(11):883-91.

[32] Interview: Doctor Mayo Tells How to Live, Better Homes & Gardens, 1934

[33] Mattila KJ, Nieminen MS, Valtonen VV, Rasi VP, Kesaniemi YA, Syrjala SL, Jungell PS, Isoluoma M, Hietaniemi K, Jokinen MJ. Association between dental health and acute myocardial infarction. BMJ 1989 Mar 25;298(6676):779-81.

[34] Osterberg T, Mellstrom D, Sundh V. Dental health and functional 'ageing'. A study of 70-year-old people. Community Dent Oral Epidemiol 1990 Dec;18(6):313-8.

[35] Evans, B. Dictionary of Quotations, Bonanza Books, p. 702.

[36] CDC/NCHS ICD-9 Categories 390-398, 402, 404-429 Death Maps. 1988-92.

[37] Mencken, H. L. A New Dictionary of Quotations from Ancient & Modern Sources. Alfred A. Knopf, Inc. Publisher. p. 126.

[38] Genesis 2:7, New Living Translation Bible. Tyndale House Publishers

[39] Enlow D.H., Hans. M. G. Essentials of Facial Growth. W.B. Saunders Company. 1996.

[40] Yamada T, Tanne K, Miyamoto K, Yamauchi K. Influences of nasal respiratory obstruction on craniofacial growth in young Macaca fuscata monkeys. Am J Orthod Dentofacial Orthop. 1997 Jan;111(1):38-43.

[41] Wright JL. Diseases of the small airways. Lung 2001;179(6):375-96.

[42] McGill HC Jr, McMahan CA, Herderick EE, Zieske AW, Malcom GT, Tracy RE, Strong JP. Obesity accelerates the progression of coronary atherosclerosis in young men. Circulation 2002 Jun 11;105(23):2712-8.

[43] Do KL, Ferreyra H, Healy JF, Davidson TM. Does tongue size differ between patients with and without sleep disordered breathing? Laryngoscope 2000 Sep;110(9):1552-5.

[44] Kimmelman CP. The systemic effects of nasal obstruction. Otolaryngol Clin North Am 1989 Apr;22(2):461-6.

[45] Lundberg JO, Farkas-Szallasi T, Weitzberg E, Rinder J, Lidholm J, Anggaard A, Hokfelt T, Lundberg JM, Alving K. High nitric oxide production in human paranasal sinuses. Nat Med 1995 Apr;1(4):370-3.

[46] Issa A, Lappalainen U, Kleinman M, Bry K, Hallman M. Inhaled nitric oxide decreases hyperoxia-induced surfactant abnormality in preterm rabbits. Pediatr Res 1999 Feb;45(2):247-54.

[47] Schedin U, Norman M, Gustafsson LE, Herin P, Frostell C. Endogenous nitric oxide in the upper airways of healthy newborn infants. Pediatr Res 1996 Jul;40(1):148-51.

[48] McCann SM, Licinio J, Wong ML, Yu WH, Karanth S, Rettorri V. The nitric oxide hypothesis of aging. Exp Gerontol 1998 Nov-Dec;33(7-8):813-26.

[49] Lundberg JO, Settergren G, Gelinder S, Lundberg JM, Alving K, Weitzberg E. Inhalation of nasally derived nitric oxide modulates pulmonary function in humans. Acta Physiol Scand 1996 Dec;158(4):343-7.

[50] Albert J, Schedin U, Lindqvist M, Melcher A, Hjemdahl P, Frostell C. Blockade of endogenous nitric oxide production results in moderate hypertension, reducing sympathetic activity and shortening bleeding time in healthy volunteers. Acta Anaesthesiol Scand 1997 Oct;41(9):1104-13.

[51] Gray LP. Results of 310 cases of rapid maxillary expansion selected for medical

reasons. J Laryngol Otol 1975 Jun;89(6):601-14.

[52] Mencken, H. L. A New Dictionary of Quotations from Ancient & Modern Sources. Alfred A. Knopf, Inc. Publisher. p. 281.

[53] Alon US. Nocturnal enuresis. Pediatr Nephol 1995 Feb;9(1):94-103.

[54] Moulden A. Management of bedwetting. Aust Fam Physician 2002 Feb;31(2):161-3.

[55] Hamburger B. Treating nocturnal enuresis. Can Nurse 1993 Apr;89(4):26-8.

[56] Schulpen TW. The burden of nocturnal enuresis. Acta Paediatr 1997 Sep;86(9):981-4.

[57] Gouda H, Cochat P, Cavailles ML, Said MH. Enuresis and benign micturition disorders in childhood. II. Cost of management. Arch Pediatr 1995 Jan;2(1):65-9.

[58] Schmitt BD. Nocturnal enuresis. Pediatr Rev 1997 Jun;18(6):183-90; quiz 91.

[59] Pugner K, Holmes J. Nocturnal enuresis: economic impacts and self-esteem preliminary research results. Scand J Urol Nephrol Suppl 1997;183:65-9.

[60] Glicklich LB. An historical account of enuresis. Pediatrics 1951.

[61] Rogers J. Nocturnal enuresis should not be ignored. Nurs Stand 1998 Nov 18-24;13(9):35-8.

[62] Noorgaard JP, Djurhuus JC. The pathophysiology of enuresis in children and young adults. Clin Pediatr (Phila) 1993 Jul;Spec No:5-9.

[63] Gimpel GA, Warzak WJ, Kuhn BR, Walburn JN. Clinical perspectives in primary nocturnal enuresis. Clin Pediatr (Phila) 1998 Jan;37(1):23-9.

[64] Robson WL, Jackson HP, Blackhurst D, Leung AK. Enuresis in children with attention-deficit hyperactivity disorder. South Med J, 1997 May;90(5):503-5.

[65] Schaefer CE, DiGeronimo TF, Toilet Training Without Tears, Signet Publisher, Revised Edition 1997.

[66] Tietjen DN, Husmann DA. Nocturnal enuresis: a guide to evaluation and treatment. Mayo Clin Proc 1996 Sep;71(9):857-62.

[67] Norgaard JP, Djurhuus JC. The pathophysiology of enuresis in children and young adults. Clin Pediatr (Phila) 1993 Jul;Spec No:5-9.

[68] Gimpel GA, Warzak WJ, Kuhn BR, Walburn JN. Clinical perspectives in primary nocturnal enuresis. Clin Pediatr (Phila) 1998 Jan;37(1):23-9.

[69] Maizels M, Gandhi K, Keating B, Rosenbaum D. Diagnosis and treatment for children who cannot control urination. Curr Probl Pediatr 1993 Nov-Dec;23(10):402-50.

[70] Thompson S, Rey JM. Functional enuresis: is demopressin the answer? J Am Acad Child Adolesc Psychiatry 1995 Mar;34(3):266-71.

[71] Donoghue MB, Latimer ME, Pillsbury HL, Hertzog JH. Hyponatremic seizure in a child using desmopressin for nocturnal enuresis. Arch Pediatr Adolesc Med 1998 Mar;152(3):290-2.

[72] Alon US. Nocturnal enuresis. Pediatr Nephrol 1995 Jun;9(3):94-103.

[73] Rey JM, Bird KD, Hensley VR. Bedwetting and psychopathology in adolescents. J Paediatr Child Health, 1995 Dec;31(6):508-12.

[74] Timms DJ. Rapid maxillary expansion in the treatment of nocturnal enuresis. Angle Orthod 1990 Fall;60(3):229-33; discussion 234.

[75] Kurol J, Modin H, Bjerkhoel A. Orthodontic maxillary expansion and its effect on nocturnal enuresis. Angle Orthod 1998 Jun;68(3):225-32.

[76] Timms DJ. Rapid maxillary expansion in the treatment of nocturnal enuresis. Angle Orthod 1990 Fall;60(3):229-33; discussion 234.

[77] Kurol J, Modin H, Bjerkhoel A. Orthodontic maxillary expansion and its effect

on nocturnal enuresis. Angle Orthod 1998 Jun;68(3):225-32.

[78] Weider DJ, Hauri PJ. Nocturnal enuresis in children with upper airway obstruction. Int J Pediatr Otorhinolaryngol 1985 Jul;9(2):173-82.

[79] Ng DK, Chau KW, Kwok KL. Nocturnal enuresis and obstructive sleep apnoea in two children. Singapore Med J 2001 Dec;42(12):590-1.

[80] Enlow D.H. Handbook of Facial Growth, Saunders, 1982.

[81] Davis DW, Bell PA. Infant feeding practices and occlusal outcomes: a longitudinal study. J Can Dent Assoc 1991 Jul;57(7):593-4.

[82] Larsson E. Orthodontic aspects on feeding of young children. 1. A comparison between Swedish and Norwegian-Sami Children. Swed Dent J 1998;22(3):117-21.

[83] Paunio P, Rautava P, Sillanpaa M. The Finnish family competence Study: the effects of living conditions on sucking habits in 3-year-old Finnish children and the association between these habits and dental occlusion. Acta Odontol Scand 1993 Feb;51(1):23-9.

[84] Mortensen EL, Michaelsen KF, Sanders SA, Reinisch JM. The association between duration of breastfeeding and adult intelligence. JAMA 2002 May 8;287(18):2365-71.

[85] Ten Great Public Health Achievements in the 20th Century. Morbidity and Mortality Weekly Report. April 02, 1999 48(12);241-243.

[86] Wahl MJ. Amalgam—Resurrection and redemption. Part 1: the clinical and legal mythology of anti-amalgam. Quintessence Int 2001 Jul-Aug;32(7):525-35.

[87] Bengtsson C, Ahlqwist M, Beergdahl IA, Lapidus L, Schutz A. No connection between the number of amalgam fillings and health. Epidemiological observations from a population study of women in Gothenburg. *Lakartidningen* 2001 Feb 28;98(9):930-3.

[88] Mjor IA, Moorhead JE. Selection of restorative materials, reasons for replacement, and longevity of restorations in Florida. J Am Coll Dent 1998 Fall;65(3):27-33.

[89] http://www.clinicians.org/RxDemos/MedProb.html.

[90] Lubbe J, Wothrich B. Amalgam allergy and amalgam controversy. Schweiz Med Wochenschr 1996 Apr 20;126(16):661-5.

[91] Stromberg R, Langworth S, Soderman E. Mercury inductions in persons with subjective symptoms alleged to dental amalgam fillings. Eur J Oral Sci 1999 Jun;107(3):208-14.

[92] Ahlqwist M, Bengtsson C, Lapidus L. Number of amalgam fillings in relation to cardiovascular disease, diabetes, cancer and early death in Swedish women. Community Dent Oral Epidemiol 1993 Feb;21(1):40-4.

[93] American Dental Association Council on Scientific Affairs. Dental amalgam: update on safety concerns. J Am Dent Assoc 1998 Apr;129(4):494-503.

[94] McComb D. Occupational exposure to mercury in dentistry and dentist mortality. J Can Dent Assoc 1997 May;63(5):372-6.

[95] American Dental Association. Code of Ethics: 5.A.1. Dental Amalgam.

[96] Odom JG. Ethics and dental amalgam removal. J Am Dent Assoc 1991 Jun;122(7):69-71.

[97] Wirz J, Ivanovic D, Schmidli F. Mercury loading from amalgam fillings. Schweiz Monatsschr Zahnmed 1990;100(11):1292-8.

[98] Bailer J, Rist F, Rudolf A, Staehle HJ, Eickholz P, Triebig G, Bader M, Pfeifer U. Adverse health effects related to mercury exposure from dental amalgam fillings: toxicological or psychological causes? Psychol Med 2001 Feb;31(2):255-63.

[99] Furhoff AK, Tomson Y, Ilie M, Bagedahl-Strindlund M, Larsson KS, Sandborgh-Englund G, Torstenson B, Wretlind K. A multidisciplinary clinical study of patients suffering from illness associated with release of mercury from dental restorations. Medical and odontological aspects. Scand J Pim Health Care 1998 Dec;16(4):247-52.

[100] Soderholm KJ, Mariotti A. BIS-GMA —based resins in dentistry:are they safe? J Am Dent Assoc 1999 Feb;130(2):201-9.

[101] Tang AT, Bjorkman L, Ekstrand J. New filling materials —an occupational health hazard. Ann R Australas Coll Dent Surg 2000 Oct;15:102-5.

[102] Lazarou J, Pomeranz BH, Corey PN. Incidence of adverse drug reactions in hospitalized patients: a meta-analysis of prospective studies. JAMA 1998 Apr 15;279(15):1200-5.

[103] Johnson JA, Bootman JL. Drug-related morbidity and mortality. A cost-of-illness model. Arch Intern Med 1995 Oct 9;155(18):1949-56.

[104] Carossa S, Bucca C, De Lillo A, Corsalini M, Rizzatti A, Lombardo S, Pera P. Correlation between edentulism, sleep disorders and arterial hypertension. Preliminary research. Minerva Stomatol 2000 Sep;49(9):399-404.

[105] Ibid.

[106] Mencken, H. L. A New Dictionary of Quotations from Ancient & Modern Sources. Alfred A. Knopf, Inc. Publisher. p. 775.

[107] Ibid. p. 775.

[108] Price, Weston A. Nutrition and Physical Degeneration. Keats Publishing, Inc. and Price-Pottenger Nutrition Foundation. 1939.

[109] Kempf HG, Roller R, Muhlbradt L. Correlation between inner ear disorders and temporomandibular joint diseases. HNO 1993 Jan;41(1):7-10.

[110] Morgan DH, Goode RL, Christiansen RL, Tiner LW. The TMJ-ear connection. Cranio 1995 Jan;13(1):42-3.

[111] Fosarelli P, Wilson M, De Angelis C. Prescription medications in infancy and childhood. Am J Dis Child 1987 Jul;141(7):772-5.

[112] Gungor A, Bluestone CD. Antibiotic theory in otitis media. Curr Allergy Asthma Rep 2001 Jul;1(4):364-72.

[113] Bluestone C.D., Stool S.E., Kenna M.A. Pediatric Otolaryngology. Volume one. 3rd edition. W.B. Saunders. 1996.

[114] Li WC, Chiu NC, Hsu CH, Lee KS, Hwang HK, Huang FY. Pathogens in the middle ear effusion of children with persistent otitis media: implications of drug resistance and complications. J Microbiol Immunol Infect 2001 Sep;34(3):190-4.

[115] Bluestone C.D., Klein J.O. Otitis Media in Infants and Children. 2nd ed. Philadelphia. WB Saunders. 1995.

[116] NIH Pub. No. 97-4216, NIDCD on Otitis Media, May 1997.

[117] Hinton, A, Herdman RC, Hartley C, O'Keefe L. The incidence of bacteria in middle ear effusions. Clin Otolaryngol 1996 Apr;21(2):158-61.

[118] Ballenger J.J., Snow J.B. Otorhinolaryngology Head and Neck Surgery. Fifteenth Edition. Williams & Wilkins. 1996.

[119] Labro MT. Antibiotics as anti-inflammatory agents. Burr Opin Investig Drugs. 2002 Jan;3(1):61-8.

[120] Burling S: Germ City. What if children's earaches were caused, not by individual bacteria, but by a whole community of them banded together to fight off antibiotics? It's the latest theory. The Philadelphia Inquirer, 2/2/98.

[121] Ballenger J.J., Snow J.B. Otorhinolaryngology Head and Neck Surgery. Fif-

teenth Edition. Williams & Wilkins. 1996.

[122] Bubon MS. Documented instance of restored conductive hearing loss. Funct Orthod 1995 Jan-Feb;12(1):26-9.

[123] Tilyard MW, Dovey SM, Walker SA. Otitis media treatment in New Zealand general practice. NZ Med J 1997 Apr;110(1042):143-5.

[124] Lazarou J, Pomeranz BH, Corey PN. Incidence of adverse drug reactions in hospitalized patients: a meta-analysis of prospective studies. JAMA 1998 Apr 15;279(15):1200-5.

[125] Moore, Thomas J., George Washington Univ., Prescription Drug Dangers, Bottom Line Personal Interview, June 1, 1998.

[126] NIH Pub. No. 97-4216, NIDCD on Otitis Media, 1997.

[127] McDonnell JP, Needleman HL, Charchut S, Allred EN, Roberson DW, Kenna MA, Jones D. The relationship between dental overbite and eustachian tube dysfunction. Laryngoscope 2001 Feb;111(2):310-6.

[128] Loudon ME. Recent advancements in vertical dimension: primary molar build-ups. Funct Orthod 1990 Jan-Feb;7(1):10-1,13-7.

[129] Page DC. FJO: functional jaw orthopedics, dental targeted treatments, medical "co-incidental" results. Funct Ortho 1988 Jan-Feb;5(1):12-7,21.

[130] Interview: Knickman E, DVM, Veterinarian

[131] Jackson JM, Mourino AP. Pacifier use and otitis media in infants twelve months of age or younger. Pediatr Dent 1999 Jul-Aug;21(4):255-60.

[132] Niemela M, Uhari M, Mottonen M. A pacifier increases the risk of recurrent acute otitis media in children in day care centers. Pediatrics 1995 Nov;96: 884-8.

[133] Branam SR, Mourino AP. Minimizing otitis media by manipulating the primary dental occlusion: case report. J Clin Pediatr Dent 1998 Spring;22(3):203-6.

[134] Cooper BC, Cooper DL, Lucente FE. Electromyography of masticatory muscles in craniomandibular disorders. Laryngoscope 1991 Feb;101(2):150-7.

[135] Lawrence HP, Garcia RI, Essick GK, Hawkins R, Krall EA, Spiro A 3rd, Vokonas PS, Kong L, King T, Koch GG. A longitudinal study of the association between tooth loss and age-related hearing loss. Spec Care Dentist 2001 Jul-Aug;21(4):129-40.

[136] Bjorne A, Agerberg G. Craniomandibular disorders in patients with Meniere's disease: a controlled study. J Orofac Pain 1966 Winter;10(1):28-37.

[137] Nomura M, Motegi E, Isoyama Y, Tochikura M, Ogiuchi H, Sepata M. Case report lateral cross bite. Part I Mixed dentition. Bull Tokyo Dent Coll 1995 May;36(2):91-7.

[138] Van der Linden, Frans P.G.M. Facial Growth and Facial Orthopedics. Quintessence Publishing Co. 1986.

[139] The New Webster's Comprehensive Dictionary of the English Language. American International Press. 1985 p. BT-83.

[140] Rubin RM. Facial deformity: a preventable disease? Angle Orthod 1979 Apr;49(2):98-103.

[141] Van der Linden, Frans P.G.M. Facial Growth and Facial Orthopedics. Quintessence Publishing Co. 1986.

[142] www.headaches.org National Headache Foundation.

[143] World Health Organization, Headache 2000 Report.

[144] www.migraines.org M.A.G.N.U.M., Migraine Awareness Group.

[145] Lamey PJ, Steele JG, Aitchison T. Migraine: the effect of acrylic appliance design on clinical response. Br Dent J 1996 Feb 24;180(4):137-40.

[146] www.headaches.org National Headache Foundation.

[147] Diane Sawyer, ABC News, Good Morning America, 9/5/01.

[148] Packard RC. Epidemiology and pathogenisis of posttraumatic headache. J Head Trauma Rehab 1999 Feb;14(1):9-21.

[149] Mattila KJ, Nieminen MS, Valtonen VV, Rasi VP, Kesaniemi YA, Syrjala SL, Jungell PS, Isoluoma M, Hietaniemi K, Jokinen MJ. Association between dental health and acute myocardial infarction. BMJ 1989 Mar 25;298(6676):779-81.

[150] Mattila KJ, Valtonen VV, Nieminen M, Et al. Dental infection and the risk of new coronary events; prospective study of patients with documented coronary artery disease. Clin Infect Dis 1995 20(3):588-592.

[151] Hamasha AA, Hand JS, Levy SM. Medical conditions associated with missing teeth and edentulism in the institutionalized elderly. Spec Care Dentist 1998 May-Jun;18(3):123-7.

[152] Loesche WJ. Periodontal disease; link to cardiovascular disease. Compend Contin Educ Dent 2000 Jun;21(6):463-6.

[153] Deaths: Preliminary data for 2000. National vital statistics reports. CDC Volume 49. Number 12.

[154] State-specific mortality from sudden cardiac death—United States, 1999. MMWR Morb Mortal Wkly Rep 2002 Feb 15;51(6):123-6.

[155] Takata Y, Ansai T, Matsumura K, Awano S, Hamasaki T, Sonoki K, Kusaba A, Akifusa S, Takehara T. Relationship between tooth loss and electrocardiographic abnormalities in octogenarians. J Dent Res 2001 Jul;80(7):1648-52.

[156] Mandel ID. Oral infections: impact on human health, well-being, and health-care costs. Compend Contin Educ Dent 2002 May;23 (5):403-13.

[157] Budtz-Jorgensen E, Chung JP, Rapin CH. Nutrition and oral health. Best Pract Res Clin Gastroenterol 2001 Dec;15(6):885-96.

[158] www.CDC.gov. Frequently Asked Questions: Complete Tooth Loss.

[159] Matilla KJ. Dental infections as a risk factor for acute myocardial infarction. Eur Heart J 1993 Dec;14 Suppl K:51-3.

[160] Matilla KJ, Valtonen VV, Nieminen MS, Asikainen S. Role of infection as a risk factor for atherosclerosis, myocardial infarction , and stroke. Clin Infect Dis 1998 Mar;26(3):719-34.

[161] Hujoel PP, Drangsholt M, Spiekerman C, DeRouen TA. Periodontal disease and coronary disease risk. JAMA 2000 Sep 20;284(11):1406-10.

[162] Azuma Y, Maehara K, Tokunaga T, Hashimoto M, Ieoka K, Sakagami H. Systemic effects of the occlusal destruction in guinea pigs. In Vivo 1999 Nov-Dec;13(6):519-24.

[163] Hescot P, Bourgeois D, Doury J. Oral health in 35-44 year old adults in France. Int Dent J 1997 Apr;47(2):94-9.

[164] Czukor J. WHO epidemiologic studies in Hungary in 1985 and 1991. Forgorv SZ 1994 Aug;87(8):223-35.

[165] Artaud-Wild SM, Connor SL, Sexton G, Connor WE. Differences in coronary mortality can be explained by differences in cholesterol and saturated fat intakes in 40 countries but not in France and Finland. A paradox. Circulation 1993 Dec;88(6):2771-9.

[166] Vargane HP, Adany R. Trends of premature mortality from cardiovascular diseases in Hungary and the European Union, 1970-1997. Orv Hetil 2000 Mar 19;141(12):601-7.

[167] McGeveran, William A. The World Almanac and Book of Facts. 2002.

[168] Mencken, H. L. A New Dictionary of Quotations from Ancient & Modern Sources. Alfred A. Knopf, Inc. Publisher. p. 294.

[169] Interview: Douglass R, CeqDT, Equine Dentist.

[170] Greene CS. The etiology of temporomandibular disorders: implications for treatment. J Orofac Pain 2001 Spring;15(2):93-105;discussion 106-16.

[171] www.pro-equinedentistry.com/skullbluelabeled2.htm.

[172] Interview: Shoemake L., Equine Professional

[173] A few definitions: Equine Dentistry: www.wellwellwell.com/newfiles/definitions.htm.

[174] Voronin IM, Belov AM, Chuchalin AG. Obstructive sleep apnea in patients with stage I arterial hypertension. Ter Arkh 2001;73(3):51-5.

[175] Silverberg DS, Iaina A, Ocksenberg A. Sleep-related breathing disturbances: their pathogenesis and potential interest to the nephrologist. Nephrol Dial Transplant 1997 April;12(4):680-3.

[176] Wofford MR, King DS, Wyatt SB, Jones DW. Secondary Hypertension: Detection and Management for the Primary Care Provider. J Clin Hypertens (Greenwich) 2000 Mar;2(2):124-131.

[177] Roux F, D'Ambrosio C, Mohsenin V. Sleep-related breathing disorders and cardiovascular disease. Am J Med 2000 Apr 1;108(5):396-402.

[178] Fritsch K, Bloch KE. Noninvasive alternatives to CPAP in therapy of obstructive sleep apnea syndrome. Ther Umsch 2000 Jul;57(7):449-53.

[179] Findley LJ, Levinson MP, Bonnie RJ. Driving performance and automobile accidents in patients with sleep apnea. Clin Chest Med 1992 Sep;13(3):427-35.

[180] Findley LJ, Unverzagt ME, Suratt PM. Automobile accidents involving patients with obstructive sleep apnea. Am Rev Respir Dis 1988 Aug;138(2):337-40.

[181] Elliot WJ. Cyclic and circadian variations in cardiovascular events. Am J Hypertens 2001 Sep;14(9 Pt 2):291S-295S.

[182] Interview: Members of Jacksonville, MD. Volunteer Fire Dept.

[183] Mehta A, Qian J, Petocz P, Darendeliler MA, Cistulli PA. A randomized, controlled study of a mandibular advancement splint for obstructive sleep apnea. Am J Respir Crit Care Med 2001 May;163(6):1457-61.

[184] Lowe AA, Sjoholm TT, Ryan CF, Fleetham JA, Ferguson KA, Remmers JE. Treatment, airway and compliance effects of a titratable oral appliance. Sleep 2000 Jun 15;23 Suppl 4:S172-8.

[185] American Academy of Pediatrics. Pediatric Pulmonology, Subcommittee on Obstructive Sleep Apnea Syndrome. Pediatrics 2002.

[186] Kim JS, Song WH, Shin C, Park CG, Seo HS, Shim WJ, Oh DJ, Ryu SH, Rho YM. The prevalence and awareness of hypertension and relationship between hypertension and snoring in the Korean population. Korean J Intern Med 2001 Jun;16(2):62-8.

[187] Racionero Casero MA, Garcia Rio F, Pino Garcia JM, Prados Sanchez C, Lobato S, Villamor Leon J. The sleep apnea syndrome as a health problem. An estimation of its prevalence and morbimortality. An Med Interna 1999 Feb;16(2):97-102.

[188] Ip MS, Lam B, Ng MM, Lam WK, Tsang KW, Lam KS. Obstructive sleep apnea is independently associated with insulin resistance. Am J Respir Crit Care Med 2002 Mar 1;165(5):670-6.

[189] Meng Q, Wang J, Wang Z, et Al. A study on the risk factors of cerebral infarction as complication of type 2 diabetes mellitus patients. Zhonghua Liu Xing Bing

Xue Za Zhi 2001 Jun;22(3):208-11.

[190] Corbo GM, Forastiere F, Agabiti N, Pistelli R, Dell'Orco V, Perucci CA, Valente S. Snoring in 9 to 15 year-old children: risk factors and clinical relevance. Pediatrics 2001 Nov;108(5):1149-54.

[191] Gozal D, Pope DW Jr. Snoring during early childhood and academic performance at ages thirteen to fourteen years. Pediatrics 2001 Jun;107(6):1394-9.

[192] Skevas A, Karamberis S, Barlamis G, Sklavounou-Tsoyrouktsoglou S. Cor pulmonale due to upper airway obstruction by hypertrophied tonsils and adenoids. Laryngol Rhinol Otol (Stuttg) 1978 Sep;57(9):804-7.

[193] Brodsky L, Moore L, Stanievich JF. A comparison of tonsillar size and oropharyngeal dimensions in children with obstructive adenotonsillar hypertrophy. Int J Pediatr Otorhinolaryngol 1987 Aug;13(2):149-56.

[194] Sasamura Y, Kudo F. Study of the effects of adenoid-tonsillar operation in infants under 2 years of age. Nippon Jibiinkoka Gakkai Kaiho 1999 Sep;102(9):1022-7.

[195] Gozal D. Sleep-disordered breathing and school performance in children. Pediatrics 1998 Sep;102(3 Pt1):616-20.

[196] Oulis CJ, Vadiakas GP, Ekonomides J, Dratsa J. The effect of hypertrophic adenoids and tonsils on the development of posterior crossbite and oral habits. J Clin Pediatr Dent 1994 Spring;18(3):197-201.

[197] Yonkers AJ, Spaur RC. Upper airway obstruction and the pharyngeal lymphoid tissue. Otolaryngol Clin North Am 1987 May;20(2):235-9.

[198] Robinson AC, Hanif J, Dumbreck LA, Prichard AJ, Manners BT. Throat swabs in chronic tonsillitis: a time-honoured practice best forgotten. Br J Clin Pract 1997 Apr-May;51(3):138-9.

[199] Kurien M, Stanis A, Job A, Brahmadathan, Thomas K. Throat swab in the chronic tonsillitis: how reliable and valid is it? Singapore Med J 2000 Jul;41(7):324-6.

[200] Ying MD. Immunological basis of indications for tonsillectomy and adenoidectomy. Acta Otolaryngol Suppl 1988;454:279-85.

[201] Wong HB. The problems of tonsils and adenoids. J Singapore Paediatr Soc 1989;31(3-4):97-102.

[202] Lind MG, Lundell BP. Tonsillar hyperplasia in children. A cause of obstructive sleep apneas, CO_2 retention, and retarded growth. Arch Otolaryngol 1982 Oct;108(10):650-4.

[203] Tal A, Leiberman A, Margulis G, Sofer S. Ventricular dysfunction in children with obstructive sleep apnea:radionuclide assessment. Pediatr Pulmonol 1988;4(3):139-43.

[204] Brown OE, Manning SC, Ridenour B. Cor pulmonale secondary to tonsillar and adenoidal hypertrophy: management considerations. Int J Pediatr Otorhinolaryngol 1988 Nov;16(2):131-9.

[205] Connick CM, Fos PJ, Barsley RE. Gender differences in special needs populations. Dent Clin North Am 2001 Jul;45(3):541-53.

[206] Vigild M. Periodontal conditions in mentally retarded children. Community Dent Oral Epidemio 1985 Jun;13(3):180-2.

[207] Schuster G, Giese R. Retrospective clinical investigation of the impact of early treatment of children with Down's syndrome according to Castillo-Morales. J Orofac Orthop 2001 Jul;62(4):255-63.

[208] Smith DS. Health care management of adults with Down syndrome. Am Fam

Physician 2001 Sep 15;64(6):1031-8.

[209] Yoshida K. Elastic retracted oral appliance to treat sleep apnea in mentally impaired patients and patients with neuromuscular disabilities. J Prosthet Dent 1999 Feb;81(2):196-201.

[210] Levanon A, Tarasiuk A, Tal A. Sleep characteristics in children with Down syndrome. J Pediatr 1999 Jun;134(6):755-60.

[211] Enlow D.H., Hans. M. G. Essentials of Facial Growth. W.B. Saunders Company. 1996.

[212] Zhao Y, YeD. Measurement of biting force of normal teeth at different ages. Hua Xi Yi Ke Da Xue Xue Bao 1994 Dec;25(4):414-7.

[213] The Baltimore Sun Paper. Dear Abby. Grinding one's teeth can lead to trouble. Universal Press Syndicate. January 28, 1988.

[214] Page DC. The orthodontic shift towards functional jaw orthopedics. Funct Orthod 2000 Oct-Dec;17(4):14-7.

[215] Schellhas KP, Piper MA, Omlie MR. Facial skeleton remodeling due to temporomandibular joint degeneration: an imaging study of 100 patients. ANJR Am J Neuroradiol 1990 May;11(3):541-51.

[216] Page DC. FJO: functional jaw orthopedics, dental targeted treatments, medical "co-incidental" results. Funct Orthod 1988 Jan-Feb;5(1):12-7, 21.

[217] Stangl DP. A cephalometric analysis of six Twin Block patients. A study of mandibular (body and ramus) growth and development. Funct Orthod 1997 Mar-Apr;14(2):4-6,8-14,17-9.

[218] Lautrou A, Salvadori A. Growth and choices in orthopedic and orthodontic therapy. Orthod Fr 2000 Dec;71(4):325-34.

[219] Turgeon-O'Brien H, Lachapelle D, Gagnon PF, Larocque I, Maheu-Robert LF. Nutritive and nonnutritive sucking habits: a review. ASDC J Dent Child 1996 Sep-Oct;63(5):321-7.

[220] Hornell A, Aarts C, Kylberg E, Hofvander Y, Gebre-Medhin M. Breastfeeding patterns in exclusively breastfed infants: a longitudinal prospective study in Uppsala, Sweden. Acta Paediatr 1999 Feb;88(12):1412-3.

[221] Setchell KD, Zimmer-Nechemias L, Cai J, Heubi JE. Exposure of infants to phyto-estorgens from soy-based infant formula. Lancet 1997 Jul 5;350(9070):23-7.

[222] Fort P, Moses N, Fasano M, Goldberg T, Lifshitz F. Breast and soy-formula feedings in early infancy and the prevalence of autoimmune thyroid disease in children. J Am Coll Nutr 1990 Apr;9(2):164-7.

[223] Moore SE, Cole TJ, Collinson AC, Poskitt EM, McGregor IA, Prentice AM. Prenatal or early postnatal events predict infectious deaths in young adulthood in rural Africa. Int J Epidemiol 1999 Dec;28(6):1088-95.

[224] Frankel S, Elwood P, Sweetnam P, Yarnell J, Smith GD. Birth weight, body-mass index in middle age, and incident coronary heart disease. Lancet 1996 Nov 30;348(9040):1478-80.

[225] Jensen TK, Toppari J, Keiding H, Skakkebaek NE. Do environmental estrogens contribute to the decline in male reproductive health? Clin Chem 1995 Dec;41(12 Pt 2):1896-901.

[226] Setchell KD, Zimmer-Nechemias L, Cai J, Heubi JE. Exposure of infants to phyto-estrogens from soy-based infant formula. Lancet,1997 Jul 5;350(9070):23-7.

[227] Beischer NA, De Garis CN. Unexplained intrauterine death near term. Aust N Z J Obstet Gynaecol 1986 May;26(2):99-101.

[228] Lefcourt LA, Rodis JF. Obstructive sleep apnea in pregnancy. Obstet Gynecol

Surv 1996 Aug;51(8):503-6.
[229] Feinsilver SH, Hertz G. Respiration during sleep in pregnancy. Clin Chest Med 1992 Dec;13(4):637-44.
[230] Schoem SR. Oral appliances for the treatment of snoring and obstructive sleep apnea. Otolaryngol Head Neck Surg 2000 Feb;122(2):259-62.
[231] Franklin KA, Holmgren PA, Jonsson F, Poromaa N, Stenlund H, Svanborg E. Snoring, pregnancy-induced hypertension, and growth retardation of the fetus. Chest 2000 Jan;117(1):137-41.
[232] Feinsilver SH, Hertz G. Respiration during sleep in pregnancy. Clin Chest Med 1992 Dec;13(4):637-44.
[233] Gray LP. Septal manipulation in the neonate: method and results. Int J Pediatr Otorhinolaryngol 1985 Mar;8(3):195-209.
[234] Page DC. Breastfeeding is early functional jaw orthopedics (an introduction). Funct Orthod 2001 Fall;18(3):24-7.
[235] U.S. Surgeon General Breastfeeding Guidelines. www.4women.gov
[236] Beaudry M, Dufour R, Marcoux S. Relation between infant feeding and infections during the first six months of life. J Pediatr 1995 Feb;126(2):191-7.
[237] Saarinen UM, Kajosaari M. Breastfeeding as prophylaxis against atopic disease: prospective follow-up study until 17 years old. Lancet 1995 Oct 21;346(8982):1065-9.
[238] Black, R. F., Jarman, L., Simpson, J. The Support Of Breastfeeding. Jones and Bartlett Publishers, 1998, Page 11.
[239] Page DC. Breastfeeding is early functional jaw orthopedics (an introduction). Funct Orthod 2001 Fall;18(3):24-7.
[240] Beaudry M, Dufour R, Marcoux S. Relation between infant feeding and infections during the first six months of life. J Pediatr 1995 Feb;126(2):191-7.
[241] www.infactcanada.ca/whocode and www.ibfan.org.
[242] Van der Linden, Frans P.G.M. Facial Growth and Facial Orthopedics. Quintessence Publishing Co. 1986.
[243] Ahlin J. H., White G. E., Tsamtsouris A., Saadia M. Maxillofacial Orthopedics: A Clinical Approach for the Growing Child. 1984.
[244] Aarts C, Hornell A, Kylberg E, Hofvander Y, Gebre-Medhin M. Breastfeeding patterns in relation to thumb sucking and pacifier use. Pediatrics 1999 Oct;104(4):e50.
[245] Pugh LC, Milligan RA, Frick KD, Spatz D, Bronner Y. Breastfeeding duration, costs, and benefits of a support program for low-income breastfeeding women. Birth 2002 Jun;29(2):95-100.
[246] Rowe-Murray HJ, Fisher JR. Baby friendly hospital practices: cesarean section is a persistent barrier to early initiation of breastfeeding. Birth 2002 Jun;29(2):124-31.
[247] Labbok MH. Health sequelae of breastfeeding for the mother. Clin Perinatol 1999 Jun;26(2):491-503, viii-ix.
[248] Davis DW, Bell PA. Infant feeding practices and occlusal outcomes: A longitudinal study. J Can Dent Assoc 1991 Jul;57(7):593-4.
[249] Farsi NM, Salama FS. Sucking habits in Saudi children: prevalence, contributing factors and effects on the primary dentition. Pediatr Dent 1997 Jan-Feb;19(1):28-33.
[250] Melsen B, Stensgaard K, Pedersen J. Sucking habits and their influence on swallowing pattern and prevalence of malocclusion. Eur J Ortho 1979;1(4):271-80.

[251] Brian Palmer, D.D.S., Presentation Research Conclusions: Ancient Skulls.

[252] Weston A. Price, D.D.S., Nutrition and Physical Degeneration, 6th edition.

[253] Kluemper GT, Beeman CS, Hicks EP. Early orthodontic treatment: what are the imperatives? J Am Dent Assoc 2000 May;131(5):613-20.

[254] Nomura M, Motegi E, Isoyama Y, Tochikura M, Ogiuchi H, Sepata M. Case report lateral cross bite. Part I Mixed dentition. Bull Tokyo Dent Coll 1995 May;36(2):91-7.

[255] Campbell PM. The dilemma of Class III treatment. Early or late? Angle Orthod 1983 Jul;53(3):175-91.

[256] Woods M. Overbite correction and sagittal changes: late mixed-dentition treatment effects. Aust Orthod J 2001 Nov;17(2)2:69-80.

[257] Nomura M, Motegi E, Isoyama Y, Tochikura M, Ogiuchi H, Sepata M. Case report lateral cross bite. Part I Mixed dentition. Bull Tokyo Dent Coll 1995 May;36(2):91-7.

[258] www.braces.org/braces/about/faq/faq_background.cfm.

[259] Luyten C. Guided tooth eruption via serial extraction. Rev Belge Med Dent 1995;50(2):67-78.

[260] Evans, B. Dictionary of Quotations, Bonanza Books, 1968. p. 702.
Miguel de Cervantes:Don Quixoti, 1605

[261] Tonetti MS. Cigarette smoking and periodontal diseases: etiology and management of disease. Ann Periodontol 1998 Jul;3(1):88-101.

[262] Muller HP. Smoking and periodontal health. Gesundheitswesen 2000 Jul;62(7):400-8.

[263] Osterberg T, Mellstrom D, Sundh V. Dental health and functional 'ageing'. A study of 70-year-old people. Community Dent Oral Epidemiol 1990 Dec;18(6):313-8.

[264] Matilla KJ, Nieminen MS, Valtonen VV, Rasi VP, Kesaniemi YA, Syrjala SL, Jungell PS, Isoluoma M, Hietaniemi K, Jokinen MJ. Association between dental health and acute myocardial infarction. BMJ 1989 Mar 25;298(6676):779-81.

[265] Osterberg T, Mellstrom D, Sundh V. Dental health and functional "ageing". A study of 70 year old people. Community Dent Oral Epidemiol. 1990 Dec;18(6):313-8.

[266] Page DC, FJO: functional jaw orthopedics, dental targeted treatments, medical "co-incidental" results. Funct Ortho 1988 Jan-Feb;5(1):12-7,21.

[267] Kempf HG, Roller R, Muhlbradt L. Correlation between inner ear disorders and temporomandibular disease. HNO 1993 Jan;41(1):7-10.

[268] Saffer M, Lubianca Neto JF, Piltcher OB, Petrillo VF. Chronic secretory otitis media: negative bacteriology. Acta Otolaryngol 1996 Nov;116(6):836-9.

[269] Branam SR, Mourino AP. Minimizing otitis media by manipulating the primary dental occlusion: case report. J Clin Pediatr Dent 1998 Spring;22(3):203-6.

[270] Timms DJ. Rapid maxillary expansion in the treatment of nocturnal enuresis. Angle Orthod Fall 1990;60(3):229-33; discussion on 234.

[271] Barthlen GM, Brown LK, Wiland MR, Sadeh JS, Patwari J, Zimmerman M. Comparison of three oral appliances for treatment of severe obstructive sleep apnea syndrome. Sleep Med 2000 Oct 1;1(4):299-305.

[272] Goldberg R. Treatment of obstructive sleep apnea, other than with continuous positive airway pressure. Curr Opin Pulm Med 2000 Nov;6(6):496-500.

[273] Fritsch K, Bloch KE. Noninvasive alternatives to CPAP in therapy of obstructive sleep apnea syndrome. Ther Unsch 2000 Jul;57(7):449-53.

[274] Page DC. The new dental-medical renaissance. Medically efficacious functional jaw orthopedics. Funct Orthod 1999 Jan-Mar;16(1):16-22,24-5.

[275] Gray. LP. Results of 310 cases of rapid maxillary expansion selected for medical reasons. J Laryngol Otol 1975 Jun;89(6):601-14.

[276] The New Webster's Comprehensive Dictionary of the English Language. American International Press. 1985 p. BT-93.

[277] Bradley, J.P., Daniels, L.F., Jones, T.C. (1975). International Encyclopedia of Quotations, J. G. Ferguson Publishing Company. p. 734.

[278] Health and Human Services Department's Centers for Medicare and Medicaid Services Report.

[279] Palmer C. Health care spending up: economists say stability 'coming to an end.' ADA News 33(2):1,25, January 21, 2002.

[280] Bodane C, Brownson K. The growing acceptance of complementary and alternative medicine. Health Care Manag (Frederick) 2002 Mar;20(3):11-21.

[281] Oral Health in America: A Report of the Surgeon General. Rockville, MD: US Department of Health and Human Services, National Institute of Dental and Craniofacial Research, National Institutes of Health, 2000.

[282] Mandel ID. Oral Infections" Impact on Human Health, Well-Being, and Health-Care Costs. Compend Contin Educ Dent. 2002 May;23(5):403-6.

[283] Altman DG. Poor-quality medical research: what can journals do? JAMA 2002 Jun 5;287(21):2765-7.

[284] Kempers RD. Ethical issues in biomedical publications. Fertil Steril 2002 May;77(5):883-8.

[285] Dickersin K, Min YI. Publication bias: the problem that won't go away. Ann N Y Acad Sci 1993 Dec 31;703:135-56; discussion 146-8.

[286] H. Berton McCauley, D.D.S. Past President, American Academy of the History of Dentistry, Journal of the History of Dentistry, 1998

[287] American Dental Association, ADA News, February 18, 2002, page 1.

[288] American Dental Association, The ADA Principles of Ethics and Code of Professional Conduct: 5.A.2. Unsubstantiated Representations.

[289] The New Webster's Comprehensive Dictionary of the English Language. American International Press. 1985 p. BT-80.

"The Wounded of Gettysburg"
U.S. Field Hospitals at Gettysburg
July 1st – 3rd, 1863

"No written nor expressed language could ever picture the field of Gettysburg! Blood! Blood! And tattered flesh! Shattered bones and mangled forms almost without the resemblance of human beings! Faces torn and bruised and lacerated…groans and cries, moans and **grinding teeth!**"

—**Army Surgeon,** *who operated on some of the 27,000 wounded involved in furious combat at Gettysburg.*

This Book and other health education products
are available at *special quantity discounts*
for bulk purchases
for healthcare patient education,
for sharing with family and friends,
for fund raising, for company giveaways,
for educational use and for book resellers.

For details, write or telephone Special Sales at ...

SmilePage^{SM} Publishing
PO Box 20300
Baltimore, MD 21284

1-410-296-7224

or visit SmilePage^{SM} Publishing online at...

www.SmilePage.com

Some special purchase options are on page 160.

SmilePage^{SM} Publishing *Quick Order Form*

	Fax Orders:	*Fax This Form Toll Free to:* **1-888-865-JAWS**
🖷	Web Orders:	**www.SmilePage.com**
🕾	Phone Orders:	1-410-296-7224 (*Have Credit Card Ready*)
✉	Postal Orders:	SmilePage^{SM} Publishing
		PO Box 20300
		Baltimore, Maryland 21284 U.S.A.

EDUCATIONAL PRODUCTS	#	Price	Total
Your Jaws~Your Life *Hardcover Book*		$ 24.95	
Your Jaws~Your Life *Paperback Book*		$ 15.95	
Your Jaws~Your Life *Audio-Cassette (Abridged)*		$ 16.95	
Your Jaws~Your Life *Audio CD (Abridged)*		$ 17.95	
Meniere's Disease & Dental Care *VHS Video*		$ 19.95	
Nutrition and Physical Degeneration/Price *Book*		$ 19.95	
Oral Motor Assessment & Treatment/Bahr *Book*		$ 49.00	
Essentials of Facial Growth/Enlow *Book*		$ 57.00	
Maxillofacial Orthopedics.../Ahlin *Book*		$ 79.00	
10 **Functional Jaw Orthopedics** *Brochures*		$ 5.00	
10 **Primary Molar Vertical Build-up** *Brochures*		$ 5.00	
Teach Family & Friends The Great Health Reasons To Save Teeth			
Save 10% on Educational Bulk Packs			
5 Books or 5 Audio-Cassettes or 5 Audio CDs			
5 **Your Jaws~Your Life** *Paperback Books*		$ 71.77	
5 **Your Jaws~Your Life** *Audio-Cassettes (Abridged)*		$ 76.27	
5 **Your Jaws~Your Life** *Audio-CDs (Abridged)*		$ 80.77	
SUB-TOTAL (total before adding tax and shipping)	→		
Maryland Orders or Delivery Add 5% State Tax	→		
☐ **Ship in U.S. Standard**: Orders $1-99.00 add $5.00, $100-199 add $10, $200-500 add $20, Over $500 we add.	→		
☐ **Ship in U.S. Priority (2-4 days)** (rates vary greatly) ☐ **Ship International Standard (4-6 weeks)** (rates vary) ☐ **Ship International Priority (3-14 days)** (rates vary)	Cost will be added. →		
TOTAL ORDER (total due with tax and shipping)	→		

PAYMENT METHOD: ☐MasterCard ☐Visa ☐Check Enclosed

Credit Card#:_____

Name on Card:_____ Exp. Date:___/___/___

Card Holder Signature:_____

Phone: ( )_____ Fax: ( )_____

Contact Person: Email:

SHIP TO:_____